REMEDIABLE ARTERIAL DISEASE

REMEDIABLE ARTERIAL DISEASE

ROY H. CLAUSS, M.D.

Professor of Surgery
New York Medical College

WALTER REDISCH, M.D.

Visiting Professor of Medicine and Research Surgery
New York Medical College

Illustrations by **Philip Johnson**
Former Assistant Professor of Surgery, Medical Illustrator
New York University School of Medicine

Grune & Stratton   *New York and London*

The cover design was adapted by
ANITA DUNCAN
from the "Fallen Man" series of etchings by
PIERRE JAQUEMON,
with the permission of the artist.

Grune & Stratton, Inc.
111 Fifth Avenue, New York, New York 10003

Library of Congress Catalog Card Number   76-157447

International Standard Book Number   0-8089-0724-7

Printed in the United States of America (G-Ho)

FOREWORD

As vascular surgery has developed during the past quarter century, there have been many major advances in diagnostic procedures and in therapeutic methods. During the last decade a number of books by vascular surgeons have been published which vary in nature from comprehensive texts to operative manuals for the neophyte vascular surgeon. As might be expected, most of these tend to be heavily biased from the surgical viewpoint.

Dr. Clauss has contributed richly to the surgical aspects of the book, having had substantial experience in the field—during the past two decades either as a resident or staff surgeon at Peter Bent Brigham Hospital in Boston, Columbia Presbyterian Medical Center, New York University Medical Center, and most recently Flower and Fifth Avenue Hospital in New York. As a reflection of the current nature of the text, the bibliography reflects mainly the major contributions appearing in the North American literature during the past year. The text is well organized, easy to read, and nicely illustrated. The roentgenograms and technical drawings emphasize clinical aspects of particular value to the resident surgeon or young practitioner, who is still "less than the best" and by virtue of more or less satisfactory training is often given the responsibility for the proper management of vascular problems in the community. Dr. Clauss provides "mini" teaching exercises in his legends, and in the diagrams he aims at correcting simple but frequently observed technical faults. He provides a philosophy and logic as well as objective indications for choosing certain forms of surgical treatment, including reconstructive surgery, sympathectomy, and amputation.

This approach emanates from his close collaboration with his co-author, who has added basic information to the text providing a fuller understanding of the pathophysiology involved in remediable arterial disease. Dr. Redisch's discussion of arterial circulation includes an updated and practical consideration of the microcirculation, a field of significant interest to him for more than forty years. In addition, he provides a medical assessment of the nonsurgical measures and drugs available for patients in whom reconstructive surgery is not feasible.

This book is a valuable addition to the resources available to physicians concerned with arterial disease and is one of the few that has substantial usefulness for student and graduate, surgeon and internist.

June 1, 1971

RALPH A. DETERLING, JR., M.D.
*Professor and Chairman, Department of Surgery,
Tufts University School of Medicine, and Surgeon-in-Chief,
New England Medical Center Hospitals, Boston, Massachusetts;
President, International Cardiovascular Society*

v

PREFACE

Review of fifteen years of personal and recorded experience with vascular surgery suggests that much of the progress made and still to be achieved is due to formulation of correct concepts and practice of precise techniques. This book presents physiologic and practical viewpoints of surgeon and internist devoting specialty interest to the study of patients with vascular disease. It is intended to provide practicing physicians, students, and house staff members bases for judgments in their care of patients. It encourages consideration of the many manifestations of ischemia and urges systematic, informed examination. Subtler phases of detection and evaluation are explained, for example, blood flow responses to exercise, serial angiography.

Most of the angiograms portray information we consider revealing, emphasizing the spirit of learning and the concept of better care through serial angiography. Preoperatively, this pathophysiologic evaluation seeks remediable new causes (e.g., ulcerated plaques) or unsuspected or associated conditions. At operation and soon after, physicians and patients should want proof of expected accomplishment or, failing this, prompt recognition of incomplete correction or iatrogenic pathology. Awareness of faults of current techniques is essential to discover the need to alter practices, be they as dramatic as avoiding application of vascular clamps or as simple as precise placement of sutures.

Arterial trauma has not been given special mention. While atherosclerotic lesions in the wall of arteries are the focus of the book, the role of microcirculation and the consequences of abnormalities of plasma and formed elements are acknowledged. The nature and significance of microvascular disease, largely an unappreciated entity, are described. Now the difference is known between micro-angiitic ulcerations, to be treated systemically, and gangrenous lesions due to arterial occlusion, to be treated by reconstructive surgery. Distinctions between venous, arterial, and microvessel type thromboses and the various sources and effects of embolization are important.

The conservative management of occlusive arterial disease had been a sad chapter in medicine for hundreds of years. In the hope that the same may not be said of surgical treatment, and that continuing advances will be recorded, it is encouraging to observe the progress in physiologic study of peripheral blood flow, defining objectively pertinent parameters of the circulation.

Incorrect practices of overlooked diagnosis, needless concern, and dilatory treatment with ineffective drugs are contrasted with propitious approaches to therapy. Manifestations of severe systemic disease in multiple locations are *not* categoric contraindications to appropriate management. Physiologic monitoring abets good judgment and precise technique in meeting challenges related to indicated surgical reconstructive procedures. We consider failures following vascular surgery to be the consequences of faults in teaching, learning, selection, performance, and evaluation. This volume does not duplicate descriptive articles and atlases which abound, but tries to convey to all readers (and especially learning and practicing surgeons) those essential details required for predictable success. It is hoped the extensive captions complement the excellent drawings of Philip Johnson, communicating essence and detail.

The selection of bibliography primarily from the 1970 literature was intended to encourage readers to peruse these readily accessible, recently published articles. The many authors who first described topics of others' more recent reports are asked to tolerate this reasoning. Generally these newer works creditably complement their books and articles with extensive references, so that neither originators of concepts nor readers of this volume will suffer from the limited but current bibliography appended to each chapter.

We gratefully acknowledge our many teachers, past and present, whether they started us in scientific medicine or taught us to apply it better. Though unnamed they will never be forgotten. We are grateful to our local and international co-workers. We thank those who have supported and made possible our work, giving encouragement in words, deeds, facilities, and funds: the old New York University Research Division at Goldwater Memorial Hospital, the Departments of Surgery and Medicine and the Rheumatic Disease Study Group at New York University, the Departments of Surgery and Pharmacology and the Diabetes Research Group at the New York Medical College, the National Institutes of Health, The John A. Hartford Foundation, Inc., and other philanthropy, and our publisher, Dr. Henry Stratton and his dedicated, talented, and helpful staff. The tireless enthusiastic retyping of many drafts by Mrs. Louise Holt, Miss Catherine Harkins, and Miss Joyce Tourigny gave new status to the position of secretary, ennobling it. Both authors agree there was another, Pamela Clauss, whose indefatigable contributions led the book to consummation.

It is hoped that this book transmits a practical synthesis of knowledge from a serious study of circulatory physiology with a reasoned advocacy of forthright preventive, diagnostic, and therapeutic measures.

ROY H. CLAUSS
WALTER REDISCH

CONTENTS

REMEDIABLE ARTERIAL DISEASE

CHAPTER 1

PHYSIOLOGY OF PERIPHERAL BLOOD FLOW

NORMAL FLOW

FLOW THROUGH ARTERIES

Blood is a nonhomogeneous suspension which flows freely through normal arteries. The volume and velocity of blood flow through these channels depend upon pressure, heart rate, and resistance. Pressure is the resultant effect of force of cardiac ejection, caliber and location of the perfused arteries, and peripheral resistance. The ejected volume is absorbed by the capacity of the microchannels in the various vascular beds.

FLOW THROUGH MICROCHANNELS

The composition of the blood plays a significant role in flow through micro-channels. Poiseuille's law, which applies to flow through large arteries, is not pertinent here. The average capillary lumen equals the diameter of a single red blood corpuscle. The blood is no longer a free-flowing suspension, and factors of plasma flow predominate. There are considerable differences in plasma/red cell ratios between small and large channels. The microhematocrit, determined by lancet prick from the fingertip or earlobe, yields the whole body hematocrit, which is only 88 to 92 percent of large vessel hematocrit, demonstrating this increase in plasma volume in the microcirculation. Blood viscosity depends upon the hematocrit and the plasma globulin fraction. Changes in viscosity with red cell concentration are nonlinear. Viscosity changes affect total resistance minimally at the point of transition from macro- to microcirculation.

1

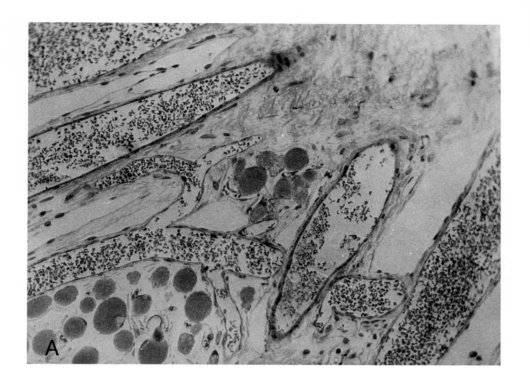

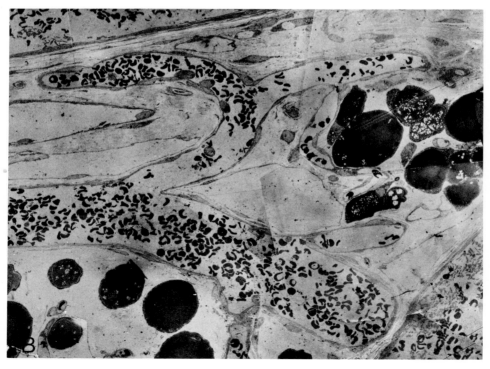

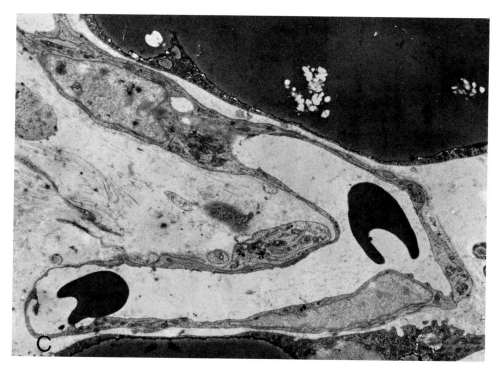

Figure 1-1. RABBIT SKIN. Longitudinal section of capillaries and venules. (A) X280; (B) X500; (C) X4,500; all figures reduced 25 percent. (*From* Rhodin, J. A. G. Ultrastructure of mammalian venous capillaries, venules, and small collecting veins. *J. Ultrastruct. Res.*, 25:452. New York, Academic Press, Inc., 1968.)

Flow Through Veins

Flow through venous channels depends mainly upon gradient between source and destination (*vis a tergo* is distinctly secondary to *vis a fronte*). Pressure, volume, and velocity of flow in peripheral veins are related to structure. Veins are "capacitance" vessels capable of accommodating large volumes of blood by passive distention. Their capability of active vasomotion is limited.

Ultrastructure

Those who attempt to integrate physiology, pharmacology, anatomy, and microcirculation are aware of the necessity for better knowledge of the untrastructure of the circulatory system.

The light microscope has not yielded sufficient magnification and resolution to make distinctions readily visible by electron microscopy (and doubtless functionally important). The electron microscope permits recognition, for example, of a wall thickness of 2000 Ångstroms from that of 500Å thickness next to it, while the light microscope shows no difference between the two. It may easily be

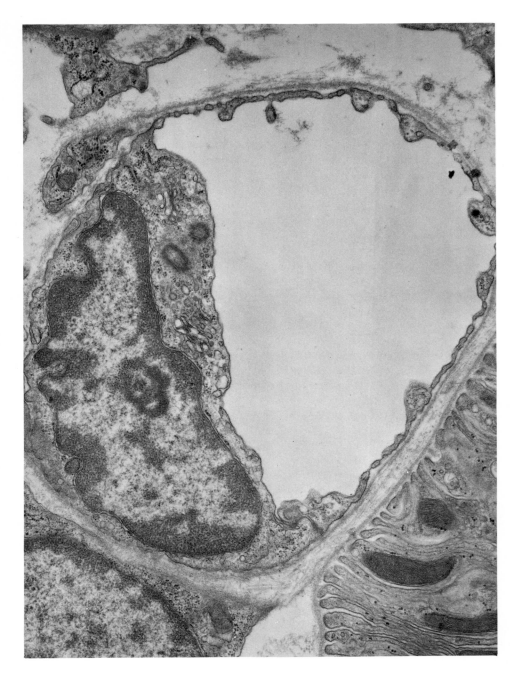

Figure 1-2. RAT KIDNEY. Cross-section through a peritubular capillary. X20,000. (*From* Rhodin, J. A. G. Fine structures of capillaries. *In* Bucklin, G. D., ed. *Topics in the Study of Life.* New York, Harper & Row, Publishers, 1970, p. 220.)

seen how this applies to the analysis of complex ultrastructures and their correlation to physiologic, pharmacologic, and biochemical changes.

Dr. Johannes A. G. Rhodin has used a particularly ingenious technique of pinpointing specific ultrastructures (e.g., precapillary sphincters), and analyzing the same anatomical site by proceeding to higher and higher magnifications (Figs. 1-1 and 1-2).

ABNORMAL FLOW

ATHEROSCLEROSIS AND OTHER OCCLUSIVE VASCULAR DISEASE

Atherosclerosis and other occlusive arterial diseases are pathologic processes affecting the arterial segment, causing diminished supply of arterial blood, with privation of nutrients and oxygen. Pain, pallor, decreased surface temperature, and trophic changes ensue. Tissue necrosis (usually called gangrene where the extremities are concerned) occurs whenever the arterial blood supply to the part is critically impaired or totally obstructed.

Atherosclerosis is a diffuse process with clinical manifestations occurring most frequently in patients above the age of 50, but it is not uncommon in persons between 30 and 45 years old and is occasionally seen in patients in their twenties. Progressive thickening of the arterial wall occurs with or· without calcium deposition.

In our experience, about 95 percent of occlusive arterial diseases are due to the development of atherosclerotic plaques with secondary thrombus formation, leading to stenosis of the involved artery. This stenosis commonly remains constant for many years, but it may lead rapidly toward complete occlusion of the vessel. General factors (e.g., dehydration, hypotension, reduced cardiac output, changes within the coagulation mechanism) or local events (e.g., injury, subendothelial hemorrhage) may precipitate occlusions and sequelae of curtailed arterial flow.

Acute arterial occlusion refers to incidents in which the main arterial supply to the part is interrupted suddenly. Symptomatology may be instantaneous, but more often it develops within minutes to an hour, depending upon the organs rendered ischemic. In the extremities, the presenting complaints are coldness (subjective and objective), pallor, and numbness. The pallor soon gives way to a mottled cadaverous appearance and the numbness to intense pain; the affected part of the limb becomes extremely sensitive even to light touch, then anesthetic.

Acute vascular insufficiency can cause gradations of ischemia, being less severe when well-developed and functional collateral circulatory pathways exist. Multiple lesions in arteries in sequence magnify ischemic symptoms and sequelae.

Favorable anatomy or site of obstruction may permit acute episodes to appear chronic, eliciting evidences of vascular insufficiency only in response to functional demand. There are limits to arterial reserve, affected by individual variations in collateral circulation, site and circumstances of arterial obstruction, and responses to measures intended to enhance blood flow.

Five percent of patients with occlusive disease have various forms of endangiitis, a progressive endothelial proliferation of unknown etiology. Obliteration of lumina of arteries of the aortic arch and upper extremities in young and middle-aged women was classified as "primary arteritis" and has been called "pulseless disease." A similar type of occlusive disease is also seen in men. A 74-year-old male with typical aortic syndrome which none of the observers doubted to be of atherosclerotic etiology was shown at autopsy to have proliferating endangiitis. A small percentage of men with Leriche syndrome have the above-mentioned mysterious endangiitis.

An entity probably belonging to the group of sensitivity angiitis, autogenous and/or exogenous, has been described as periarteritis nodosa, recently more appropriately called polyarteritis nodosa. The main location of the lesions is in the arterioles and in the microvasculature, although this type of generalized angiitis does affect arterial vessels.

About one out of five instances of nonatherosclerotic arterial occlusion (less than one percent of all arterial occlusive disease) is due to thromboangiitis obliterans, as described by von Winiwarter in 1879 and later popularized by Buerger. It is characterized by (1) proved relationship to tobacco sensitivity, (2) appearance of superficial phlebitis as a clinical precursor of the arterial involvement, (3) early involvement of upper extremity arteries, and (4) specific microscopic features. It was said to be a disease of young men who had been heavy smokers since youth; however, the disease has been described in women also. Ethnic specificity in Jews has been disproved. It is true that this erroneous diagnosis has been made far too frequently when the process was actually occlusive atherosclerosis, but thromboangiitis obliterans does exist as an uncommon form of occlusive disease.

Instances of so-called "toxic arteritis" are rare. The best-substantiated type in this small group of angiitides is the necrotizing obliterative endarteriitis observed in ergot poisoning. There was a noticeable increase in incidence of this malady when ergotamine-tartrate injections were used too freely to abort attacks of migraine headaches. Ergot gangrene attacks fingers and toes predominantly, starting always at the tips. Ergot endangiitis can easily be demonstrated experimentally in the tail of the rat. Recently another drug, methysergide (Sansert), used to allay cluster headaches, has been proved damaging to the vascular system in some patients. Retroperitoneal fibrosis and fibrotic stenoses and occlusions in the aorta and its larger branches have been observed.

Bacteremias, especially subacute and acute bacterial endocarditis, are prone to produce embolic phenomena. At times such septic emboli may be large enough to lodge within a large or medium-sized artery and lead to the development of a mycotic aneurysm.

Complete occlusion of an arterial channel need not be entirely organic; functional and pharmacologic constriction may preclude blood flow. Spasm per se —that is, pathologic local constriction in a perfectly healthy artery—probably never occurs except in Raynaud's phenomenon, where the local peripheral syncope of arteriolar channels has been proved to be brought about by stimuli exerted upon an abnormally sensitive sympathetic nervous system. Even in this instance, the possibility of preformed structural abnormalities of digital arteries is still under debate. It is impossible to affect complete constriction of an artery in animal experiments without previously damaging the arterial wall.

MICROVESSEL PATHOLOGY

Interference with proper function of the minute circulation affects metabolic exchange through the capillary wall and may lead to increased capillary permeability, local edema, diminution or loss of capillary tonus, hemorrhage, and even necrosis. Some angiitides show no arterial changes initially; they are called "microangiitides" and can be visualized best by surface capillaroscopy.

Microvascular derangement has been recognized for some time as characteristic of rheumatic disease. Some of the changes have been observed to be constant and predictable, and may be considered to represent typical patterns of disease processes in rheumatoid arthritis, systemic lupus erythematosus, scleroderma, and progressive systemic sclerosis. However, these changes may not be interpreted as pathognomonic. They merely serve as useful parameters of analysis of microcirculation just as accepted hemodynamic criteria are used to analyze macrocirculation.

Raynaud's phenomenon (attacks of peripheral syncope) has no distinctive microcirculatory findings in the absence of clinical evidence of sclerodermatous changes.

Ischemic ulcerations may be found in rheumatoid disorders in the proved absence of occlusive arterial disease. Progression of ulceration depends upon the course of the basic disease. While morphologic and flow changes found in capillaries of skin and mucous membrane cannot be proved to exist simultaneously in viscera, it seems certain that the minute vessels respond systemically and not just locally.

Recent advances in x-ray equipment and angiographic techniques will provide further approaches to the investigation of microcirculation. Microangiography has been used to study microvascular patterns in biopsy and postmortem tissues of muscle, brain, and lung. Current research methods of microangiography permit visualization of arterioles (30 to 300μ) but employ unacceptable exposure to radiation for use in human beings.

INFLAMMATION

All observers expect a visibly inflamed area to have a discernibly increased temperature relative to surrounding surfaces, even in ischemic extremities. Measurements made in markedly ischemic extremities which exhibit inflammation disclose flow values equal to normal resting quantities. Intra-arterial injection of potent anticonstrictor substances increases flow still more. These phenomena encourage the speculation that inflammation is a stimulus evoking increased perfusion into the extremity through grossly inadequate conduit channels; this far exceeds the amount of blood induced to flow prior to the onset of inflammation. Locally, quantities of perfusion in response to inflammation have been estimated at 50 times normal. As already noted, if flow through the conduit channels is elevated only to normal, necrosis, not healing, will occur. The provocative thesis containing hope for patients with such ischemic yet inflamed extremities is that a way may be found to retain the stimulus to increased flow while controlling the incitants and the destructive effects of inflammation, causing the latter to subside (e.g., antibiotics, systemic and local medical-surgical treatment). Among the reasons for nonhealing following amputation is the belief that surgical trauma invokes just as great a demand for nutrients and effluence of metabolites as necrosis does. This is far in excess of stimulated flow.

The two main vascular beds of the extremity are located in the skin and in the muscle (ignoring the practically immeasurable flow to bone). A physiologic example of stimulating blood flow to the skin is inducing increased heat dissipation via an extremity following forced heat accumulation in the body (Gibbon-Landis procedure). Increased metabolism of muscle is induced by exercise. In markedly ischemic extremities, the increased flow of blood attending inflammation has not been adequate for nutritional purposes, since the function of the exchange vessels is more complicated than is yet known. Blood reaching a vascular bed may serve intricate transport mechanisms with specialized local functions (e.g., immunologic), leaving little or none to serve nutritional demands in the given setting. Better knowledge of the ultrastructure of small vessels hopefully will lead to fuller understanding of their specific functional responses.

RESTORED FLOW

FLOW THROUGH ARTERIES

Measurements of blood flow before and after reconstructive surgery have been compared with the use of adrenergic blocking agents and with the effects of sympathectomy.

Normal lower extremities of adult human beings studied by venous occlusion plethysmography in constant temperature rooms at 20°C and 55 percent humidity disclosed blood flow of 4 ml/100 grams tissue per minute. In legs with occluded arteries, flow ranged between 0.5 and 2.0 ml. The Gibbon-Landis procedure was followed by increases in skin perfusion of 60 percent, with no change in muscle perfusion. Regional exercise caused slight increase of blood flow to skin but increases of 100 percent in muscle flow. Norepinephrine caused a significant decrease in both skin and muscle perfusion with normal or diseased arteries under all experimental conditions.

Eight to ten days after successful revascularization procedures, blood flow measurements were normal. After sympathectomy, skin perfusion was significantly higher, but muscle flow was unchanged. The Gibbon-Landis test caused 30 percent decrease in skin perfusion and a slight decrease in muscle perfusion. Regional exercise elicited a smaller increase in muscle flow. Systemic arterial pressure (measured at the brachial artery) remained unaltered throughout all experiments. Thus, the alteration in responses cannot be explained by a borrowing-lending phenomenon within the limb. Decrease in perfusion in both skin and muscle caused by norepinephrine was invariably magnified after sympathectomy. This exaggerated response to the most important physiologic vasoconstrictor in the internal milieu represents an especially undesirable result of sympathectomy.

In endoangiitis, the progressive narrowing and obliteration of distal arteries of medium and small caliber prohibits attempts at surgical reconstruction.

FLOW THROUGH MICROCHANNELS

Attempts to modify pathologic changes in minute vessels and to correct disturbances in blood flow through these channels are in their early stages of trial. Three basic avenues of approach are being explored by several groups of workers at present: (1) Corticosteroids are used to treat connective tissue disease, and clinical responses to the microvessels to corticosteroids appear to be dose-dependent. (2) Alpha-adrenolytic drugs (guanethidine, phenoxybenzamine) have been used to treat progressive systemic sclerosis and scleroderma. The frequency of Raynaud's phenomenon and the capillaroscopic findings of marked narrowing of the afferent limb associated with enormous widening of the efferent limb has understandably evoked the thought that abnormal sensitivity to catecholamines may be the basis of some forms of microangiitis. (3) Low molecular weight dextran modifies microangiitis by preventing increased intraluminal aggregation of red cells with delayed dispersion of the aggregates.

BIBLIOGRAPHY

1. CASSIN, B. The evolution of scintillation scanning. *In* Freeman, L. M., and Johnson, P. M., eds. *Clinical Scintillation Scanning.* New York, Harper & Row, Publishers, 1969, pp. 3-49.
2. GUYTON, A. C. *Textbook of Medical Physiology.* Philadelphia, W. B. Saunders Company, 1966.
3. MAGGIO, E. *Microcirculation.* Springfield, Ill., Charles C Thomas, Publisher, 1965.
4. RAAB, W. *Hormonal and Neurogenic Cardiovascular Disorders.* Baltimore, The Williams & Wilkins Co., 1953.
5. REDISCH, W., MESSINA, E. J., SCHWARTZ, N. S., and CLAUSS, R. H. Microcirculation. *In* Brest, A. N., and Moyer, J. H., eds. *Cardiovascular Disorders.* Philadelphia, F. A. Davis Co., 1968, pp. 135-144.
6. ——— TANGCO, F. F., and SAUNDERS, R. L. *Peripheral Circulation in Health and Disease.* New York, Grune & Stratton, Inc., 1957.
7. RHODIN, J. A. G. Fine structure of capillaries. *In* Bucklin, G. D., ed. *Topics in the Study of Life.* New York, Harper & Row, Publishers, 1970.
8. ——— Ultrastructure of mammalian venous capillaries, venules, and small collecting veins. *J. Ultrastruct. Res.,* 25:452, 1968.
9. ——— *An Atlas of Ultrastructure.* Philadelphia, W. B. Saunders Company, 1963.
10. RICHARDS, R. L. *The Peripheral Circulation in Health and Disease.* Baltimore, The Williams & Wilkins Co., 1946.
11. SHEPHERD, J. T. *Physiology of the Circulation in Human Limbs in Health and Disease.* Philadelphia, W. B. Saunders Company, 1963.
12. SOBOTTA, J. *Atlas of Human Anatomy, Vol. 3,* McMurrich, J. P., ed. New York, G. E. Stechert, 1936.
13. STRANDNESS, D. P. *Collateral Circulation.* Philadelphia, W. B. Saunders Company, 1969.
14. WOOD, P. *Diseases of the Heart and Circulation.* Philadelphia, J. P. Lippincott Co., 1956.

CHAPTER 2

BASIC CLINICAL PICTURES EVOLVING FROM DISTURBANCES IN PERIPHERAL BLOOD FLOW

INFLUENCES OF ARTERIAL
PATHOLOGIC ANATOMY UPON
FUNCTION OF END ORGANS

CAROTID-VERTEBRAL ARTERIES
CORONARY ARTERIES
CELIAC-MESENTERIC ARTERIES

RENAL ARTERIES
AORTA AND ILIAC ARTERIES
FEMORAL ARTERIES
POPLITEAL ARTERIES
TIBIAL AND PERONEAL ARTERIES

CONSEQUENCES OF ISCHEMIA

Blood flow is an essential mechanism of life. It depends upon pumps, conduits, and interplay between volumes and spaces, pressures and resistances. Circulation is influenced by viscosity, hydration, mechanisms of coagulation and fibrinolysis, local changes in the lumen of blood vessels (pathologic anatomy), and iatrogenic, inflammatory, and neurogenic processes.

Atherosclerosis causes lesions which can diminish caliber of arteries, limit pressure and flow, incite abnormal coagulation, affect organ function, and interfere with automaticity of microcirculation. Degrees of inadequate blood flow vary from undetectable to symptomatic, to disabling, to lethal. Each of these stages of vascular insufficiency is preventable, reversible, or compensable. The frequency, rapidity, and completeness of recovery from disabling ischemic syndromes by medical and surgical measures contrasted with the few instances of successful reversal of near-lethal processes emphasize the desirability of detecting limitation of blood flow in the early stages.

It is important to diagnose localized atherosclerotic lesions, for they are amenable to surgical treatment which restores function and relieves symptoms. The presence of diffuse atherosclerosis should not lessen physicians' determination to investigate, identify, and treat symptomatic focal pathology, for this can enhance comfort, enjoyment, and productivity of many patients' lives. Categories of symptoms in patients' histories should alert the physician to the diagnosis of arterial insufficiency. Searching physical examinations can support the suspected diagnosis, and angiograms may confirm, localize, and define pathology and indicate treatment and prognosis. Remediable lesions may be detected and corrected in ischemic, withered, fissured, infected extremities and in aged ill patients.

INFLUENCES OF ARTERIAL PATHOLOGIC ANATOMY UPON FUNCTION OF ORGANS

CAROTID-VERTEBRAL ARTERIES

Physicians and laymen charitably tolerate waning mental and physical performance in aging people, implicitly accepting decreased cerebral circulation as the basis of the change in function. This teleologic concept correlates well with current findings of the clinical research of Ingvar and Lassen[5] who demonstrated the relationship between function (primary) and circulation (secondary) of the brain. Reduced blood flow to gray matter is commensurate with diminished cerebration consequent to vascular disease, while reduced flow to white (supporting, glial) tissue goes unnoticed clinically. Alterations in regional flow concomitant with external stimulation were recorded without increase in total cerebral blood flow. Tragic functional disturbances of cerebrovascular accidents (CVA) have always implied, to layman and physician, profound reductions in blood flow to the brain.

The phenomenon of transient ischemic attacks (TIA) or recurrent, intermittent, neurologic deficit (RIND) was not assessed correctly by most physicians for the first fifty years of this century, despite Hunt's description in 1914 of pathologic anatomy consistent with a common cause.[4] He described extracranial stenoses and occlusions in carotid arteries and patent vasculature intracranially in patients whose clinical courses had been interpreted as due to focal intracranial occlusive disease. Subsequently, evidence from autopsy and angiographic investigations produced three categories of information which explain lack of precision in clinical diagnosis. Seventy-five percent of patients with symptomatic cerebrovascular insufficiency have stenotic and/or occlusive lesions at multiple sites, which may involve combinations of locations in vessels of intra- and extracranial, ipsi- and contralateral, and anterior and posterior circulations. Twenty percent of these patients have vascular occlusive lesions at "inappropriate" sites that is, sites which are not suspected from clinical history and examination. Twenty percent of patients whose histories suggest cerebrovascular disease do not have demonstrably abnormal circulation to the brain. Technical inadequacy of angiographic techniques may account for this, for the best x-ray equipment and techniques permit resolution only to 40 micra, and many nutritive small vessels are of lesser diameter.

In children and adults, clinical evidences of impaired circulation to the brain have come from psychologic and intelligence tests of patients subjected to anesthesia for surgical operation and cardiopulmonary bypass (extracorporeal circulation). Impaired memory and reason and alteration of personality appeared to be correlated with low carbon dioxide tension in arterial blood during controlled and assisted ventilation, and require months for return to measured normalcy. Up to 30 percent of patients with heart valve prostheses have experienced transient dizziness, tinnitus, parasthesias, monoparesis, etc., attributed to small emboli, whereas fewer than 5 percent have had major strokes.

These facts support our readiness to believe the brain is an end organ of exquisite sensitivity, and its malfunction displays itself in many ways. This information has preventive, diagnostic, and therapeutic usefulness clinically. Recovery from dysfunction may be complete. Transient malfunction demands early diagnosis, for unremedied consequences may be irreversible or fatal. Rehabilitation of patients with completed stroke is slow, tedious, costly, and often incomplete.

The simplest concepts of arterial pathologic anatomy are narrowing and occlusion. The lumen becomes constricted over a long period of time by atheroma, then suddenly it is obstructed by intraluminal thrombosis or by intramural hemorrhage into the plaque. Atherosclerotic plaques may become ulcerated, and fibrin, platelets, and corpuscular emboli which form on the thrombogenic surface become dislodged and obstruct intracranial arteries of the brain. In addition, semisolid content of plaques may be discharged into the lumen of the internal carotid artery. Such cholesterol-like material has been observed in retinal arteries of patients and in arteries of the brain at operation and autopsy.

The pathophysiology of stroke may be described as stenosis or occlusion with decreased cerebral blood flow; occlusion with cerebral blood flow so deficient as to cause infarction; and emboli and local ischemia, with or without infarction. The process can affect single or multiple sites, unilaterally or bilaterally. Physiologic consequences are sudden reduction of blood flow from one or more vascular lesions to foci or regions of the brain. Correlations may not always exist between lesion and functional effects.

Events in day-to-day living that may precipitate systemic reactive hypotension and symptomatic episodes of cerebrovascular insufficiency are getting out of bed, warm bath, exposure to warm environment (e.g., gardening, house-painting, kitchen activities), and inappropriate heart rate and rhythm (e.g., tachycardia of unusual exertion, bradycardia of Valsalva maneuver, heart block). Systemic or regional reductions in cerebral blood flow may be caused by marked or persistent rotation, extension, or flexion of neck (e.g., driving, spectator activity, reading, praying).

Neurologic symptoms and signs vary considerably among patients with identical anatomic lesions. Conversely, similar symptoms may be caused by intracranial and extracranial occlusive processes. The urgency of detecting symptoms of reduced blood supply through structurally abnormal vessels is the implication of identifying patients who are prone to strokes. Clinical recovery from transient ischemic attacks occurs in most instances permitting diagnostic studies and appropriate treatment before infarction of brain tissue ensues.

The importance of carotid arterial circulation is conceded, whereas that of a single vertebral artery is minimized. Neurosurgeons' experience with abrupt interruption of one internal carotid artery in adults is that profound hemiplegia occurs in 60 percent of instances. Surgical interruption of unilateral vertebral artery in the treatment of children with cyanotic congenital heart disease rarely causes neurologic deficit.

Cortical ischemic symptoms are secondary to diminished blood flow through the carotid artery and its area of distribution, causing typical unilateral sensory and motor symptoms. Characteristically the episodes are single, short, regressive, and infrequent. Vertebrobasilar deficiencies of circulation often cause progressive bilateral visual, sensory, and motor dysfunction and commonly exhibit vertigo and dysarthria.

Coronary Arteries

Coronary artery disease appears to be related to heredity, diet, and physiologic and stress factors. It is a progressive process starting soon after birth. Circulatory insufficiency in coronary arteries is suggested by pain (angina), dyspnea, and limited physical capacity (failure); it is confirmed by electrocardiographic abnormalities, altered biochemical reactions in blood samples obtained from peripheral vessels and coronary sinus, coronary angiograms, and death. The functional significance of coronary artery disease is implicit in the high mortality statistics.

Collateral circulation can develop and relieve many symptoms. Intractable angina and myocardial failure merit angiographic investigation; a single focal lesion may exist at a site remediable by arterial reconstruction in 15 percent of instances. Symptomatic lesions at multiple sites yield to operative treatment in several vessels. The influence of severity of stenoses in evoking collateral circulation was learned from coronary angiography before and after indirect myocardial revascularization procedures. When stenosis exceeded 85 percent of the lumen of a major coronary artery, angiographic evidence of induced circulation between implanted internal mammary artery and intrinsic vessels distal to stenosis was demonstrated in almost 90 percent of patients. In contrast, when stenoses occluded less than 85 percent of the lumen, fewer than half the myocardial implants in patients demonstrated flow angiographically. There was a high correlation between demonstrated blood flow and symptomatic relief.

Inadequate coronary artery circulation is compensated by anaerobic metabolism in the myocardium. Metabolic studies disclosed excessive lactic acid in blood from the coronary sinus of patients with angina pectoris due to inadequate coronary arterial flow. The lactic acid concentration was elevated further by increased heart work, and reduced when increments in myocardial blood flow were achieved.

In experimental animals, correlations have been established between mortality and acute and chronic interruption of coronary artery circulation. Focal and regional electrocardiographic assessment in dying animals indicated effects of inadequate coronary artery circulation (e.g., anaerobiosis, altered pH, potassium efflux, and cell membrane instability). Explanation of survival despite severe dysrhythmia seems more difficult. Dynamic studies controlling flow, pressure, and composition of perfusates in coronary arteries in relation to work of the heart certified once again the general concept that pathologically inadequate perfusion exerted ill-effects upon myocardial function.

Celiac-Mesenteric Arteries

Abrupt occlusions of superior mesenteric arteries (or veins) precipitate dramatic clinical symptomatology long remembered by students and practitioners. Only 15 percent of patients will survive. The severe cramping pain and hyperactive bowel sounds imply tetanic contractions, relieved only by ischemic neuropathy of motor and sensory components of the parasympathetic and sympathetic systems, and loss of contractile capability of smooth muscle of intestine. Subsequent pain and tenderness are somatic in origin, secondary to inflammatory irritation of parietal peritoneum induced by transudate and exudate from walls of bowel and mesentery. Anatomically, there may be a collateral network into the superior mesenteric artery from celiac and inferior mesenteric arteries, but physiologically, the quantity of collateral flow is too small for the active metabolic needs of tissue supplied, and may merely be sufficient to propel toxic products absorbed from ischemic segments into the general circulation, with disastrous consequences. Distally, the anatomy is that of endarterial distributions with minimal connections between arcades and nearby branches of the parent artery. Functionally, reflex vasoconstriction deprives the gut of circulation in hypovolemia and hypotension. Precise correlation of the physiology of secretion, absorption, and gland function with circulatory alterations is unknown.

Spontaneous abrupt interruption of blood flow into the celiac axis seems to be extraordinarily rare. Emboli through this channel into the splenic artery are not uncommon and the symptoms, signs, and benign consequences are so well known that they excite little concern in physicians. May it be assumed that equal numbers of emboli occlude hepatic and gastric branches, even though characteristic clinical pictures have not been described?

Physicians do not often recognize symptoms caused by chronic ischemia of superior and inferior mesenteric arteries and of the celiac axis. This is not surprising, since psychic and somatic gastrointestinal dysfunctions are so common and are improved with diet and medication. Inflammatory, ulcerative, obstructive, and spastic processes are believed responsible for most upper abdominal symptoms that occur in relation to meals.

Recently, attention has been focused upon external compression of the celiac axis as a remediable cause of an ischemic syndrome. When the celiac axis originates from the aorta at a level higher than usual, it may be compressed by ligaments of the diaphragm. Pain, aching, and distention are recurrent symptoms. Their relation to meals may not be definite, and the duration of each episode may vary. Symptoms may occur as infrequently as weekly, or may occur several times a day without relation to meals. Nausea, vomiting, and diarrhea are rare. Epigastric bruits may be detected in most patients, aiding suspicion of the correct diagnosis.

Atherosclerotic occlusions of the celiac axis may produce disabling, aching epigastric pain within 30 minutes of ingestion of a meal, lasting one to three hours. Large meals may cause more severe symptoms of longer duration. Patients develop a fear of food; the "small meal syndrome" leads to weight loss. If superior mesenteric arterial insufficiency coexists, symptoms may be more severe. Stool habits may be affected; constipation may be related to quantity and composition of intake; malabsorption may occur. In some instances, these symptoms appear following removal of abdominal aortic aneurysm. It may be presumed that borderline circulation caused by stenoses of celiac or superior mesenteric arteries previously was compensated by collateral circulation from the inferior mesenteric artery, but became insufficient subsequent to ligation of the latter.

A measure of effectiveness of collateral circulation into the bed of the inferior mesenteric artery is inferred from the lack of ill effects following its ligation. In patients with abdominal aortic aneurysms subjected to operation, inferior mesenteric arteries are ligated and divided routinely, yet the reported incidence of clinically recognizable ischemia at operation is virtually nil, and is less than two percent in the postoperative period. Clinical manifestations are pain, ileus, bloody diarrhea, and peritonitis. We have never observed the phenomenon of ischemic necrosis of colon after aneurysmectomy.

RENAL ARTERIES

Renovascular hypertension has become an accepted term implying that one category of elevated blood pressure occurs secondary to disturbed vascularity of kidneys. Current knowledge indicates there is a high correlation between hypertension and elevated concentration of renin in blood from kidneys with insufficient blood flow or pressure. In our laboratory, renin levels have been highest with renal artery occlusion (recent or chronic), less high with fibromuscular hyperplasia, and least and inconsistently elevated with atherosclerotic stenosis. Correction of the cause has been followed promptly by normal levels of renin; failure to relieve the cause sustains renin elevations. We have analyzed thoracic duct lymph and renal vein blood renin in patients with fibromuscular hyperplasia and have noted raised concentrations in both fluids, followed by normal concentrations within hours of correction of the pathologic process.

Renal artery stenoses secondary to atherosclerotic plaques have been associated with hyperplasia but are not necessarily the cause; in such instances elevated renin levels have not been observed. This suggests that stenosing lesions are not the undisputed incitants of hypertension, and normotension cannot always be expected after surgical removal of the plaques. Elevated renin levels were not recorded when a vascular stenosis was inapparent, nor were they sustained following correction of the cause. False positive reactions have not been observed, but our experience and that reported in the literature is too limited to state that false negative tests, which have not occurred, cannot occur. Correlations with other prognostic criteria in large numbers of patients need to be done. Prognostic indices of Winters[13] have disclosed the greatest validity between factors present in patients with fibromuscular hyperplasia and relief by surgical treatment. Renin tests were not done.

Extreme reductions in mean blood pressure and flow to kidneys reduce filtration, reabsorption, and excretion, as shown by abnormal pyelogram, by radioactive renogram, and by split function analyses of diminished excretion of water, sodium, chloride, and creatinine. Bilateral lesions can reduce clearance of waste products, leading to uremia. It is important to realize that glomerular filtration can be reduced by 70 percent without elevations of plasma creatinine or urea. Conversely, depression of filtration below 30 percent can cause abrupt elevations in those biochemical products on successive days, since the quantities of creatinine and urea presented to the kidney exceed filtration capacity. Temporary ischemia is inherent in the procedure of renal artery reconstruction, and the diuretic regimens (water and mannitol) may promote urine flow without adequate chemical excretion.

AORTA AND ILIAC ARTERIES

Signs of functional inadequacy of circulation through the aorta and distal arteries are due to abrupt dissipation of kinetic energy at sites of stenosis or occlusion of major vessels, curtailing distribution of blood flow locally and distally. Multiple (tandem) lesions which frequently occur along the course of vessels in one extremity sequentially diminish circulation toward the periphery, intensifying local ischemic symptoms. Occlusive lesions may occur in vessels which nourish specific muscle groups or areas of skin. Classic symptoms of circulatory insufficiency are cramping pains in muscles while walking, discomfort in extremities at rest, and changes in color, temperature, and nutrition of skin.

Thirty percent or more of the cardiac output is normally distributed distal to the renal arteries. When the abdominal aorta is occluded, entrapment of normal cardiac output into two-thirds of the normal sized vascular space elevates systolic pressure markedly and diastolic blood pressure to a lesser degree. Atherosclerotic occlusive processes obstruct the distal aorta and proximal iliac arteries in women in their forties and in men in their fifties (Leriche syndrome). This causes impotence in males despite patent hypogastric, external iliac, and distal arteries. Both sexes have back pain at rest and claudication in the buttocks, thighs, and calves during exercise. Intense local back pain follows excision of the abdominal aorta with replacement by a tubular or bifurcation graft. It is not unlikely this is ischemic pain due to sudden and permanent interruption of lumbar arteries. Customarily, this pain is attributed to traumatic arthritis or ligamentous strain following prolonged relaxation of normal curvature of spine secondary to anesthesia, or to operative trauma of pre- and paravertebral areas.

During exercise, the patient experiences claudication in the calf, thigh, and buttocks, in that order, caused by unilateral and bilateral occlusion of the common iliac artery. Collateral circulation by all routes rarely compensates sufficiently to preclude such symptoms. Measurements disclose marked reduction in intra-arterial blood pressure distal to the iliac occlusive process; blood flow is only a fraction of normal. The lesion and its symptoms constitute such typical claudication that calf symptoms which occur, despite femoral pulses, have been referred to as "iliac equivalent" disease.

Occlusion of one hypogastric artery generally causes no symptoms. Coexisting lesions may contribute to symptoms. Significant stenosis of the external iliac artery on the same side restricts blood flow of collateral vessels to muscles of the buttocks, and "hip pain" occurs with exercise. Significant stenoses of contralateral common or internal iliac arteries are likely to cause claudication in both buttocks, and may cause impotence. Surgeons are so certain of the dispensability of a single hypogastric artery that one is sacrificed as a source of autogenous graft material. Both hypogastric arteries have been ligated to reduce uterine hemorrhage, but whether this causes ischemic symptoms has not been recorded. In our experience, atherosclerotic processes in hypogastric arteries tend to be both longitudinal and circumferential. Diffuse lesions occur more often than a localized plaque at the orifice. Although the caliber of secondary and tertiary branches reduces as anticipated, thickness of atheromatous process seems not to diminish proportionately, resulting in markedly narrowed lumina. Satisfactory endarterectomy with long-term patency is difficult to achieve in hypogastric arteries.

FEMORAL ARTERIES

External iliac and common femoral artery stenoses and occlusions are highly symptomatic, causing claudication in the calf and thigh. Pressure gradients of only 20 mm Hg have been associated with significant diminution of flow. Surgical reconstruction, eliminating this small gradient, has produced marked increases in flow and relief of symptoms. If stenotic or occlusive processes coexist distally, then symptoms may merely be diminished by relief of iliac obstruction. There is an important difference between atherosclerotic segmental obstruction of the common femoral artery and occlusion of the bifurcation of a common femoral artery. In the former, collateral vessels carry blood to patent major arteries of the thigh and leg. Neither chronic nor acute interruption of both branches of the common femoral artery is likely to be compatible with limb survival if the obstructing process is not removed. Furthermore, high thigh amputations rarely heal per primam if common and profunda femoris arteries are occluded or ligated.

The profunda femoris artery is an important vessel because of the large quantity of blood it carries to popliteal and tibial vessels via collateral routes. The role of the profunda femoris artery has been appreciated more since reconstructive surgical procedures and blood flow studies have demonstrated its role. Occlusion of the profunda femoris artery only, in the presence of patent normal arteries proximally and distally, causes claudication in muscles of the thigh and buttocks. Stenosis of the profunda femoris artery (readily appreciated on angiograms, despite superimposition of its profile on common and/or superficial femoral artery) coexistent with obstruction in the superficial femoral artery can markedly limit blood flow to the periphery and cause severe ischemic symptoms and signs in calf and foot, another example of so-called "iliac equivalent" disease.

Physiologic measurements and persistent reexamination have clarified the roles of superficial femoral arteries and their relation to patency in arteries proximally and distally. Obstruction of this artery occurs most commonly at the adductor canal, beginning as a narrowing which progressively diminishes the cross-sectional area. Symptoms are uncommon unless demands for blood flow in calf muscles are pronounced, (e.g., walking up hills or stairs, swimming with flippers), or where blood supply is limited by pathology in iliac, profunda femoris, popliteal, or tibial vessels. Further progression of symptoms at later dates is characteristic, coinciding with pathologic events in anatomy and blood flow. The interval until new symptoms appear is highly variable. When thrombosis becomes superimposed upon an atheromatous plaque, obstruction suddenly and simultaneously affects not only the main vessel but one or more collateral vessels by propagation of thrombus in each direction, sealing orifices already narrowed by the plaque. Severe ischemic symptoms develop and persist. The hour and date of the event usually are readily remembered by a patient, for subsequently his capacity for exercise is reduced. He may dread claudication to the extent that he changes habits and recreation, and finds alternate methods to achieve essential tasks. If occlusion of collateral vessels and propagation of thrombus occur in stages, patients frequently are aware of the several dates on which further symptoms developed. Significant narrowing of deep femoral, popliteal, or tibial arteries intensifies the limitations of activity imposed by successive reductions in blood pressure and flow.

POPLITEAL ARTERIES

Ischemic symptoms in the leg and foot are more severe when popliteal occlusion causes them than when they are due to a proximal obstructive process. Acute occlusions (emboli, trauma) are attended by high amputation rates (65 percent in World War II). Patients with chronic occlusions frequently have "hot knees" due to increased circulation through geniculate collateral supply; the skin of the knee is warmer than that of thigh and calf.

Information readily available through angiography and improved surgical results encourage the examining physician to consider the functional anatomy of the popliteal artery. The few physicians who do examine the popliteal pulse usually palpate above the knee joint line. They all know that absence of popliteal pulse may be caused by an occluded femoral artery, but too few realize that the presence of a pulse at this level does not exclude remediable stenoses at or distal to the joint line. Bounding pulses are not uncommon immediately proximal to obstructions. Successful reconstructive operations upon popliteal arteries distal to the joint line are possible; tibial and peroneal arteries may be operated upon in the leg and circulatory continuity restored. Thus, angiography must complement physical examination.

TIBIAL AND PERONEAL ARTERIES

Anatomically, a bifurcation occurs at the distal end of a popliteal artery. The anterior tibial artery originates at a wide angle directly anteriorly and crosses the interosseous membrane. The downward continuation from the popliteal bifurcation is called the tibioperoneal trunk, which divides two or three centimeters distal to its origin into posterior tibial and peroneal arteries. Frequently both the anterior tibial artery and the tibioperoneal trunk are stenotic, causing claudication. More commonly one or two of the three main arteries are occluded for long segments, and focal stenoses exist in the other arteries. Severe pain at rest or necrotic lesions of toes, heel, or foot indicate absence of patency for the full length of any of the three vessels below the knee; there is obstruction in at least one site in each of three arteries. Digital or end-artery occlusion may accompany proximal arterial obstruction, causing gangrene. It is erroneous to estimate causes or to make arbitrary judgments concerning clinical disposition without serial angiograms.

CONSEQUENCES OF ISCHEMIA

Atrophy of calf muscles, osteoporosis of bones, loss of hair on feet and legs, thin long cuticle of nails, and loss of subcutaneous fat in pads of toes and heel are "deciduation phenomena" caused by diffuse stenoses of arteries at and distal to knee level. Minimal circulatory supply cannot nourish these structures. When trauma or infection is superimposed, circulation must be restored or the extremity must be amputated.

The skin of the foot of an ischemic extremity tends to be dry, scaly, shiny, and to have intracutaneous ecchymoses. Loss of integrity of microcirculatory

of pain in respect to the extremities involved; (2) type of onset of pain, whether insidious and progressive or sudden and sustained; (3) character of pain, be it discomfort or a complaint of varying description; (4) severity of pain, which may range from an abnormal sensation to exruciating intractability; (5) circumstances that provoke appearance of pain or exacerbate its severity—trauma, systemic disease, effort, exercise, rest, body positions, specific times, and certain climatic conditions; and (6) conditions that relieve pain—rest or exercise, heat or cold, change of position, or certain drugs. In some instances pain may be attributable to neural disturbances resulting from interferences with the blood supply to nerves. Pain due to arterial insufficiency usually is intensified by elevation of the limb and alleviated by dependency. Erythermalgia is relieved by elevation and cooling.

In some cases, the patient complains of pain at rest, often disturbing his sleep; it is relieved by getting out of bed and massaging the part or stamping on the floor. This indicates a more advanced pathologic state in the arterial system. The marked deficiency of perfusion is aggravated by the lower blood pressure and cardiac output during sleep, unaided by mechanical gradient of dependent legs. The parallel to angina of effort and angina decubitus is striking.

INTERMITTENT CLAUDICATION

This term has been widely used to denote a symptom which is pathognomonic for arterial insufficiency. The classic intermittent claudication is a cramp-like pain, usually in the calf, initiated or intensified by walking, especially if done rapidly, or by climbing upstairs, and promptly relieved by rest. The location of this pain depends upon the vessels involved. For example, occlusion of the aorta at its bifurcation (Leriche syndrome) causes localization of the phenomenon in the buttocks, while the common sites of occlusion in the adductor canal and at the popliteal branching produces pain in the calf.

SENSORY DISTURBANCES

Sensory disturbances usually associated with neurologic disorders are frequently seen in patients with arterial insufficiency disease. A burning sensation or burning pain may be the complaint of patients with such divergent disorders as occlusive atherosclerosis or erythermalgia (a vasodilator disorder associated with redness and warmth of the part, aggravated by dependency of the extremity or by application of warmth and relieved by elevation of the part and cold). The phenomenon of burning pain occurs in various kinds of dermatitides but is especially characteristic for erythermalgia.

Numbness and tingling are common complaints frequently overlooked because they are usually attributed to neurologic disturbances or are overshadowed by pain or burning sensations. They may precede pain and other signs and symptoms of sudden arterial occlusion. The old problem of whether ischemia of the peripheral nervous system may lead to peripheral neuropathy or whether the two occur independently has remained a moot question. Certainly, peripheral neuropathy in diabetic patients may be found associated with an adequate peripheral arterial system, and extensive occlusive arterial disease may be present without the signs of peripheral neuropathy.

The subjective feeling of coldness is very common in occlusive vascular disorders. The part actually may be cold to the touch, and yet there may not be any demonstrable vascular pathology. Disappearance of coldness following treatment is usually the first indication of improved circulation in patients with established arterial insufficiency.

FATIGUE

This symptom in the extremities, if related to effort and recurring persistently, may be a manifestation of inadequate perfusion or oxygenation. However, it also may be secondary to mechanical factors (e.g., flat feet, hard floors, improper height of heel of shoe). Systemic disorder or neurologic disease as a cause of fatigue must be ruled out.

DISCOLORATION

Color changes of skin of an extremity may be subtle or absent despite diminished blood flow. This is common when the arterial insufficiency has progressed slowly. Acute arterial insufficiency (embolus, thrombus) causes obvious pallor, and even a dead, marble-like appearance. Long-standing marked ischemia produces rubor, which may vary through most hues of red and blue. Diagnostic and prognostic implications are inherent in color changes, emphasizing severity of ischemia and subject to interpretation of urgency for treatment.

MICROCIRCULATORY DISEASE

Acrocyanosis may be associated with warmth but more frequently with marked coldness, yet it is rarely of real clinical significance.

Raynaud's phenomenon (peripheral syncope) often is associated with severe pain. It occurs most frequently with systemic connective tissue (collagen) diseases, in the absence of occlusive arterial or major venous disease, or, it may be seen in nervous persons in the absence of any demonstrable systemic disease.

Differential diagnosis. The physician must be familiar with the general symptomatology of systemic connective tissue and sensitivity disorders to relate yet distinguish them from what may appear to be peripheral vascular disorders. The most frequent complaints of patients with systemic diseases affecting morphology and blood flow of the minute vessels are superficial rashes, diffuse and recurrent discolorations, and tiny ulcerations of tips of fingers or toes. Not uncommonly, however, symptoms are similar to those of patients with early occlusive arterial disease—coldness of extremities, discoloration, numbness, and "pins and needles" sensation. The occurrence of Raynaud's phenomenon is about 20 percent in systemic lupus erythematosus and almost 100 percent in progressive systemic sclerosis. Pain may be present in the form of arthralgia, often not easily differentiated from muscular pain and sometimes misinterpreted as intermittent claudication. There is a known occurrence of small ischemic ulcerations in extremities in progressive systemic sclerosis, and of large ischemic ulcerations in systemic lupus erythamatosus, sensitivity angiitis, and rheumatoid and psoriatic arthritis in the absence of occlusive arterial disease. Capillary microscopy and angiography will be decisive in differential diagnosis.

VENOUS DISEASE

Differential diagnosis. Patients with varicose veins usually have mild complaints readily distinguished from arterial insufficiency. Recent or chronic phlebitis of deep veins may cause discomfort and even severe pain in the calf, intensified by prolonged standing and by walking just a few steps. There is not immediate relief by cessation of walking, but there is dramatic relief with elevation (and drainage and decompression) of the extremity. Fatigue, discoloration, tingling, and coldness appear to coincide with pooling of blood, while burning or unpleasant sensation of warmth indicate continuing inflammation in and around the walls of veins. Enlargement of the limb and changes in pigmentation and texture of skin may be caused by venous stasis or occlusion. Cough, hemoptysis, and pleuritic pain suggest the complications of pulmonary embolism.

LYMPHATIC DISEASE

Differential diagnosis. Lymph stasis may be congenital or acquired and produce "brawny" nonpitting edema and enlargement of parts or all of an extremity. Infection in an extremity with recurrent regional lymphangiitis or operative trauma not uncommonly precede acquired lymphedema. Postmastectomy lymphedema is believed to be the result of multiple factors—excision of lymph channels and nodes, scarring from trauma and subclinical infection, and venous occlusion.

PHYSICAL EXAMINATION

SIZE AND SYMMETRY

Extremities may be unequal in size in the presence of arteriovenous fistulas, the involved limb being larger than its fellow in one or more dimensions. Limbs surviving arterial occlusion without the development of gangrene usually show muscular atrophy. Vascular causes of asymmetry of limbs rarely present confusion with extravascular conditions (e.g., neurogenic wasting, neoplastic enlargement).

SKIN AND SUBCUTANEOUS TISSUES

COLOR CHANGES. *Pallor.* Pallor or blanching, like redness and cyanosis, is a very common finding in vasomotor and vascular disorders and may be the presenting manifesation. In arterial insufficiency, blanching is easily induced by elevation of an extremity, while in vasomotor disorders it may be produced by exposure.

Erythema. Erythema or redness may be seen in varying shades and patterns in both upper and lower extremities. Pallor seen with elevation of the limb persists for the first few seconds on dependency of the limb, followed by redness that deepens to the purple hue. This rubor on dependency is due to pooling of blood in the minute vessels, initially from lack of propulsion, secondarily from deficient reactivity. Nonocclusive and noninflammatory causes of erythema (e.g., cold, warmth, dependency of the part, emotional disturbances) and its localization, transience or permanence, and associated symptoms (e.g., burning, pain, coldness or warmth of the involved parts) must be considered. Purely dermatologic conditions are to be recognized.

Cyanosis. Cyanosis, a bluish, dusky discoloration of the skin results from deficient oxygenation of the blood or tissues. Generalized cyanosis occurs whenever arterial oxygen saturation is subnormal, as in states of respiratory or cardiac failure. Localized cyanosis suggests inadequate or slow circulation in the part as a result either of vasospasm or impairment of drainage with local pooling in the minute vessels. Cyanosis may occur transiently in occlusive vascular disease as part of a sequence of color changes. Persistent localized cyanosis indicates a more serious or more permanent vascular disturbance. Rapidly developing persistent cyanosis associated with coldness of the parts involved usually portends impending gangrene. Blue discoloration of venous disease is comprised of myriads of discrete dilated venous channels of many widths and lengths.

ATROPHY. Atrophy of the subcutaneous tissue may be noted in long-standing arterial insufficiency. Abnormalities of the nails (e.g., hypertrophic, stunted or deformed, brittle, lusterless) and hair (e.g., scanty, thin, lusterless, brittle) are common. Specific changes producing a tight, waxy, atrophic skin are seen in scleroderma, sclerodactylia, and in some patients who exhibit Raynaud's phenomenon with a symptomatology too vague to permit their inclusion in one of the recognized disease entities.

BLEBS. Patients with vascular disease are more prone to develop blebs and blisters following minor burns and scalds. Blistering is also common in areas with moist gangrene resulting from acute arterial occlusions. Patients with arterial disease sometime develop blebs spontaneously, which present characteristic features. They appear suddenly and develop rapidly, usually overnight, and frequently are fully developed when first noticed. Association with trauma or other causes is denied. They occur on or about the toes, ranging from one centimeter to six centimeters in diameter. The inflammatory reaction is minimal, and, except for slight itching, burning, or minimal pain, they are symptomless. The fluid content is at first clear and colorless, becoming turbid and discolored, but not frankly purulent, within 24 to 48 hours, when an area of gangrene is seen at its base. The subsequent course is that of a gangrenous lesion. Occasionally such blisters are filled with dark hemorrhagic fluid.

HEMORRHAGIC EXTRAVASATIONS. Large cutaneous bruises at pressure points are not uncommon in elderly arteriosclerotic patients; they have been called "senile purpura." Petechiae and purpura may be seen in acute thromboarteritis, poly-arteritis (periarteritis nodosa), and in embolic and thrombotic microangiopathy. Telangiectasias, which are abnormally dilated capillaries, and angiomata, which are benign vascular tumors, do not cause clinically significant disturbances in blood flow.

ULCERATIONS. Ulcerations which occur or recur following minimal trauma, which present gangrenous changes, or which show no tendency to heal despite their apparent small size must be considered "ischemic" ulcers with vascular impairment as the underlying physiopathology. "Stasis" ulcers are due to impairment of venous drainage. They are localized in the lower leg, are shallow, and exhibit granulations in spite of secondary infection. Ulcers due to minute vessel disease (microangiitis) are similar to true ischemic ulcers, and are best differentiated from these by the absence of the signs of arterial occlusive disease. Capillaroscopy establishes the etiology.

CHANGES IN SURFACE TEMPERATURE. Coldness of extremities, if bilateral and symmetrical, may be normal. Marked coldness may be an expression of a primarily neurologic rather than vascular disturbance, especially if there is associated hyperhidrosis. Bilateral and symmetrical coldness occuring transiently may be found in vasospastic disorders; similar but persistent findings occur in occlusive vascular disease, concomitantly with color changes and symptoms of vascular insufficiency. Coldness of one extremity, or parts of it, evaluated best by comparison with the other limb, is almost invariably a manifestation of vascular pathology, occlusive or vasospastic in nature.

Warmth as a localized physical finding usually implies the presence of inflammation. In obliterative vascular conditions without inflammation the involved parts are cold to the touch despite the associated finding of dependent redness or erythema, or the complaint of a burning sensation. In these cases, warmth or heat indicates an inflammatory reaction to a complicating secondary infection.

The only noninflammatory vascular disturbances exhibiting abnormal warmth in the involved parts are arteriovenous fistulas and erythermalgia. Erythermalgia is characterized by warm, red and "burning" extremities, usually bilaterally and symmetrically.

NODULES. Nodules may be seen or felt beneath the skin in patients with poly-arteritis (periarteritis nodosa). Their distribution along the course of the arteries may be of diagnostic significance, which may be established by biopsy. Nodules are seen in the skin in vascular tumor and in erythema nodosum, a sensitivity to drugs.

PERIPHERAL PULSES

It is customary to palpate for the brachial and radial pulses in the upper extremities and for the femoral, popliteal, posterior tibial, and the dorsalis pedis (or its proximal part, the anterior tibial) pulses in the lower extremities. The presence or absence of pulsation and its forcefulness are noted, together with the evaluation of sclerotic changes as ascertained by the hardness, absence of elasticity, or beading of the arterial wall. Strong pulsations indicate adequate mainstem or primary circulation at the point of its detection. This does not preclude the possibility of arterial obstruction a short distance distally. Diminution in forcefulness of a pulse previously noted to be normal is usually indicative of developing arterial obstructive pathology. Absence of pulse can be due to diminished rate of perfusion of an artery from proximal obstruction (insufficient head-pressure), to actual obliteration at the site of palpation, or to an embryologic anomaly or malformation (rare). The permanent disappearance of a previously palpable pulse is a diagnostic feature of embolic or thrombotic occlusion at or proximal to the area of examination.

The fact that a pulsation cannot be felt in an accessible artery does not mean that the channel is organically obliterated at that site of palption. While proximal intraluminal obstruction is a probable cause, diminished pulses may disappear following exercise, as the increased demands for blood flow into muscles reduces the force of perfusion distally. Vasoconstriction secondary to hypovolemia, inadequate cardiac output, operative trauma to arteries, or inappropriate use of vasoactive drugs can delete a pulse temporarily.

Arteries may be blocked regionally, but secondary or collateral channels can maintain an adequate blood supply to distal parts. An abnormally located pulsation may be felt over well-developed collateral vessels when the primary channel is obstructed. An abnormally located pulsation, associated with a thrill, bruit, and/or murmur, is a common finding of arteriovenous fistulas. Similar signs encountered over an expanding pulsatile mass are almost pathognomonic for arterial aneurysm.

SPECIAL TESTS

A great number of special tests to determine the competence or adequacy of the circulation in the extremities continue to be described in many texts on peripheral vascular disease. Some of them have been highly useful, others less so. The simplicity or complexity of the tests, and the ease or difficulty of their performance are not necessarily indices of their relative clinical usefulness. Here, various tests are classified as "essential" or "contributory"; those of limited value will be disregarded. Certain of these tests are essential observations made in the course of physical examination.

CLINICAL TESTS

ESSENTIAL TESTS. *Postural color changes.* Normal persons with unimpaired arterial circulation demonstrate slight blanching of feet on elevation which returns to normal within 10 seconds on dependency. Characteristic color changes may be produced at will in limbs with arterial insufficiency. Elevation of the leg and foot above the supine patient produces blanching of the part, best appreciated on the plantar surface of the toes and soles of the feet. When the patient sits up, with his feet at the side of the bed, return of normal color is either considerably delayed (one minute or more) or the pallor is replaced by a reddish or purplish erythema that may be diffused or mottled in appearance.

Venous filling time. One of the prominent superficial veins on the dorsum of the foot is watched carefully. With the patient in a supine position, the limb is elevated to drain the veins of blood. After emptying the selected vein, the limb is lowered to the horizontal position and the time for refilling of the selected vein is noted. Normally this takes five to fifteen seconds; a delay indicates impaired arterial inflow. Venous filling times in excess of twenty seconds have prognostic significance; incisions of feet and toes may not heal and local surgery is contra-indicated. In the presence of varicose veins, venous reflux must be obviated before the limb is lowered.

CONTRIBUTORY TESTS. *Responses to exercise—Claudication time and distance.* The patient is made to walk at a regular fast pace (120 steps per minute) or to climb a flight of stairs until pain or claudication appears. The time that elapsed or the distance walked from the start of the test to the appearance of the pain is noted as the claudication time or claudication distance. A treadmill or a physiologic bicycle has been used for the same purposes.

Color changes with exercise. The supine patient with limbs elevated is made to exercise by alternately flexing and extending ankles and toes (or wrists and fingers) forty to sixty times per minute. Blanching (plantar ischemia test) and pain increase in the presence of marked arterial insufficiency.

Postural pain. Pain, if present, accompanies the postural color changes. With elevation of the limb, gravity further depletes the already insufficient arterial blood supply to the part, causing pain as well as blanching.

LABORATORY TESTS

ESSENTIAL TESTS. *Aortography and arteriography.* Plain radiography of the extremity is virtually valueless. The presence of calcification in vascular walls may be detected, but this does not provide the examiner with information regarding the patency of these vessels, the presence or absence of obstructive pathology, or the extent of compensatory collateral channels. Precise information concerning the exact site of the obstruction may be obtained by the use of radiopaque substances, which are injected percutaneously into the artery, then visualized radiographically as they course through the various arterial branches. The substance may be injected into the aorta (aortography) or into the smaller arterial trunks (arteriography). This method is necessary for the proper assessment of possibilities of primary surgical repair. Location and extent of lesions as well as patency of distal vessels are some of the important information it yields. Various substances have been employed for this purpose; sodium diatrizoate (hypaque) and meglumine iolthalamate (conray) injection have ben found most satisfactory.

CONTRIBUTORY TESTS. *Plethysmography—Use of the constant temperature-humidity laboratory.* If the rate of venous flow from a limb or organ were to remain constant, then briefly interrupted, changes in volume of the part reflect the character of arterial inflow. Qualitatively, an increase in volume of the part implies an increase in blood flow to the part; lesser increases in volume imply relatively decreased blood flow. Quantitatively, the rate of blood flow (increase or decrease) may be determined by the rapidity or acuteness of this change in volume. Several plethysmographic methods have been devised to measure blood flow, all based on the above-mentioned principle.

To ascertain the functional significance of a clinical disturbance in peripheral blood flow, it is highly desirable to be able to test the various segments separately. Total arterial supply is judged by plethysmographic baseline measurements.

The subject is allowed to adapt to a preset temperature of 23°C in the constant temperature-humidity laboratory. Blood flow to the calf is measured by venous occlusion plethysmography. After baseline values have been ascertained, the subject exercises for a period of two minutes by rhythmic flexion and extension of the foot at a rate of one cycle per second. The subject is instructed to relax and remain motionless at the end of the exercise period. Blood flow response to the exercise is determined by plethysmographic measurements after five seconds, thirty seconds, one minute, and at one-minute intervals thereafter for a total of twenty-five minutes.

Interpretation of the exercise-response curve permits conclusions as to the optimal capacity of the muscle vasculature in the tested segment, and to the capability of muscle blood flow in the segment to resist endogenous vasoconstrictor impulses

The participation of small skeletal muscle vessels may be ascertained by this regional exercise test. The performance of the capacitance vessels (veins) can be tested with a method described by Wood.

The subject is allowed to adapt to environmental temperature in the constant temperature laboratory. A Whitney strain gauge is placed around the calf, and baseline pulsations are recorded. A pneumatic cuff is placed at the ankle and inflated to above systolic pressure. A venous congesting cuff is placed just above the knee and is inflated from 0 to 30 mm Hg by increments of 5 mm Hg. The resulting increases in volume are recorded. The data obtained are plotted, and the venous pressure-volume curve is constructed.

The interpretation is based on the fact that the venous pressure-volume curves serve to evaluate the capacitance function of the segment in question. A series of curves, ascertained under varying conditions may yield information on shifts of fluid from the extrathoracic to the intrathoracic compartments and vice-versa within the segment.

Determination of the oxygen content of peripheral blood.   The amount of oxygen extracted from blood as it passes through an extremity has been used to determine adequacy of circulation to the extremity. Oxygen consumption is determined from the difference in oxygen content of the arterial and venous bloods in the extremity ("arteriovenous difference"). The usefulness of this test is limited, as the oxygen saturation of blood is influenced by various extravascular factors, and as normal wide variation is observed in venous oxygen saturation even under constant environmental and physiologic conditions. An apparatus called the oxygen electrode seems to be much more promising when used in relation to a single variable (e.g., influence of position change upon oxygen tension in skin).

Other tests. Microangiography with a search ray and photography with the x-ray camera will probably help once these procedures have advanced from experimental trials to practical use.

Injection of a bolus of Xe_{133} into the muscle belly of the gastrocnemius has been used to determine changes in muscle flow by differences in the multi-exponentiality of clearance curves. With higher blood flow (e.g., in induced hyperemia) the disappearance curves move closer together.

Pho-gamma camera scanning is a technique for documenting distribution and rate of clearance of macroaggregated albumen labelled with radioactive iodine. Intra-arterial injection of the isotope is followed by emission of gamma rays from the limb. "Cold spots" may coincide with angiographic evidences of arterial occlusion. The rate of delay of radioactivity varies with the quantity of tracer trapped in microvasculature, the factors active in degradation of albumin molecules, and the volume of blood flow per unit of time through the extremity. Experiences with five limbs before and after arterial reconstruction suggest the worth of the method in quantitating regional distribution of blood flow as it may vary independently of mainline flow.

ANGIOGRAPHY

SURVEY

Angiography refers to the technique of visualizing arteries, veins, and lymphatics by x-ray following the injection of contrast materials. Arterial studies are advisable when acute or chronic ischemic symptoms and signs indicate the need for treatment, and where definition and localization of intravascular obstructive processes may direct the most effective therapy. Demonstrating lesions unremediable by conventional surgical therapy can be as important as showing those amenable to operation. Information gained permits inferences of urgency of instituting effective medical measures (e.g., thrombolytic, anticoagulant), the probability of symptomatic relief, or the likelihood of failure of therapy.

Angiography can influence treatment of several major disease processes: emboli, atherosclerosis, aneurysm, neoplasm, fistula. Angiography is an integral part of embolectomy (see pages 74 and 77). Extracranial and/or intracranial localization of obstructing processes may be demonstrated in patients with strokes. Ulcerating atheromata may discharge contents intraluminally or precipitate thrombosis. Remediable causes and sites of lesions in patients with hypertension and coronary artery disease may be disclosed. Arterioarterial embolization may be discerned. Amputation of limbs should be preceded by angiography, since more than 15 percent of patients with gangrene have remediable lesions of proximal arteries, and amputation can be avoided or converted to local excision rather than major ablation. Angiography may diminish between aneurysm, neoplasm, or atherosclerotic obstructive vascular processes. Angiography aids in identification of fistulas; important distinguishing characteristics between diffuse and focal varieties of arteriovenous communications influence decisions concerning therapy.

The remediable phenomena that angiography can disclose invoke a practical corollary: angiographic procedures should not be terminated until desired information is demonstrated clearly. Physician, surgeon, and radiologist come to realize that precise, clear demonstration of structure, course, and rate of flow through the vessels observed in ideal angiograms must become the routine result. Seriographic exposures disclose information concerning anatomy, collateral circulation, and flow rate likely to be missed or unappreciated on single films. Peripheral arteriograms taken following transient ischemia or drug therapy (papaverine; contrast media) may improve the clarity of demonstrated pathology and aid in evaluation of peripheral small arteries. Position of the extremity (geometry of vessels) during angiography continues to merit study to determine optimum visualization. Details of exposure and techniques of developing x-ray film are important.

Ischemic symptoms and signs that suggest a focal point of inadequate circulation are evaluated best by angiography which demonstrates both contiguous and remote vessels proximal and distal to sites of suspected pathology. A survey of the aorta and its branches and arteries of both lower extremities is considered advisable in most instances when angiography is performed to evaluate a process in one lower extremity. Far-advanced atherosclerotic lesions may exist at a distant site despite absence of symptoms, and they may preclude subsequent angiography, emphasize the need for vigorous preventive medical measures, or indicate prophylactic surgical operations (a concept that will gain in popularity and practice).

Currently it is the vogue to consider surgical operation for a patient with transient ischemic attacks of the cerebrum, or with renal artery stenoses presumed the cause of hypertension, but only rarely are prophylactic procedures performed upon arteries of the extremities. Two parallel sets of experiences influence this type of thinking. There is a relatively low rate of amputation for patients with circulatory insufficiency of extremities. However, experienced surgeons also have angiograms of many documented instances of rapid progression from arterial stenosis to occlusion with disastrous consequences, as well as elective cases of reconstruction for progressive sclerosis with excellent result. The infrequency of recommendation of such procedures seems to be based upon instances of unfavorable outcome of arterial operations in circumstances of salvage or by inexperienced surgeons.

Operations upon several (tandem) lesions in arteries of an extremity may be feasible or necessary, according to the perspective permitted by adequate angiography.

Patients with clinical symptoms or signs of ischemia in the lower extremity and a history of hypertension are entitled to have renal arteries visualized as well as those in the periphery.

Patients with above-knee amputation may have ischemic symptoms on the amputated side as well as symptoms at other locations; operative reconstruction of arteries of both the intact extremity and the amputated thigh relieve ischemia. Patients with advanced ischemic sequelae of long duration may still have remediable lesions.

Claudication may seem difficult to explain when pulses are palpable in the feet. If these pulses disappear with exercise, high grade stenosis or occlusion proximally will be demonstrated on angiograms. Thus, despite the presence of pulses, there is an organic basis for symptoms and probably a focal remediable cause, which the physician can document and relieve. *Indications* for angiography are the suspicion or presence of a disease state wherein diagnosis or treatment may require precise information. Relative *contraindications* are precarious physiologic state of the patient or history of allergy to contrast media. Infection, cellulitis, and gangrene of extremities, even lymphangitis, are *not* contraindications to angiography.

Safety of angiography is enhanced by injecting the smallest amounts of contrast substance of least toxicity into well-hydrated patients and by employing systemic or local heparinization while needles, cannulae, or catheters are in vessels. Technical skill of personnel and minimal disease in the vessel used for injection increases the success and safety of angiography. Patient comfort is obtainable through rapport with his physician, explanation and assurances before and during examination, appropriate premedication, adequate local anesthesia, flawless technique, and correct dose, concentration, and details of injection. A potent analgesic minimizes the discomfort attending injections, and soporific or tranquilizer drugs allay anxiety. Needless shaving and purgation are avoided. Extravasion of contrast medium may be treated by injecting 0.5 percent or 1 percent xylocaine into the area, without moving needle or catheter. However, local anesthesia is *never* injected into lumina of *arteries to the brain*.

REGIONAL

CEREBROVASCULAR (CAROTID-VERTEBRAL) ANGIOGRAPHY

Indications for angiography of carotid and vertebral arteries are suspected pathologic changes of vessels, brain, or contiguous areas. Aneurysm, arteriovenous malformation, tumor, trauma, and atherosclerosis are common processes for which delineation is sought by neurologist, neurosurgeon, and vascular surgeon. Percutaneous retrograde angiography of the right brachial artery visualizes subclavian, vertebral-basilar, innominate, and carotid arterial distribution extra- and intracranially. In the majority of instances contrast medium enters the aorta, demonstrating the orifice of the innominate artery. Up to 40 percent of patients receive sufficient contrast substance into the left carotid artery to permit evaluation of its extracranial course. The left vertebral artery is visualized in 10 percent of subjects consequent to injection into the right brachial artery. Left brachial injection outlines left subclavian and vertebral artery distribution, and injection into the left common carotid artery shows anatomy and flow of that artery (Fig. 3-1).

Percutaneous needle and/or cannula techniques combine the advantages of simplicity, superior contrast visualization, and safety of low concentration and quantity of opaque medium distributed selectively and regionally (Fig. 3-2).

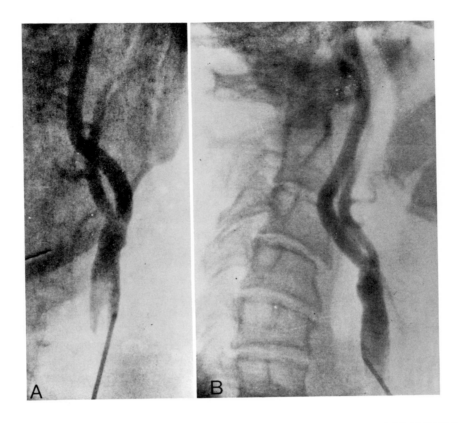

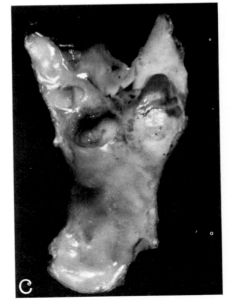

Figure 3-1. SYMPTOMATIC ULCER-ATED PLAQUE. AP and lateral views of carotid artery bifurcation disclose irregularities consistent with ulcerations of atheromatous plaques (A and B). Three ulcerations are seen in plaque (C, opened surgical specimen). This 57-year-old man with previous aorta-iliac artery reconstruction remains asymptomatic two years after carotid artery operation.

Skilled professional personnel perform procedures with local anesthesia. Insertion of needles into brachial arteries eliminates possibilities of artefacts at suspected sites of pathology, which can confuse diagnostic interpretation of x-rays or introduce pathologic processes (extravasation, dissection, hematoma; Fig. 3-3). Retrograde injection disperses contrast medium for optimal visualization, preventing nonvisualization secondary to streaming effects when contrast substance is injected in the direction of flow of blood. The needles and cannulas, in contrast to catheters, present small intraluminal foreign bodies in short segments of arteries not directly affecting cerebral circulation. They initiate spasm only locally, and present little thrombogenic surface. If reduced flow or thrombi occur, the ill effects are confined to the extremity; there is no ill effect upon cerebral circulation.

Simultaneous biplane angiography minimizes the number of injections of even small quantities of contrast substance, providing maximum three-dimensional information with least discomfort or incidence of complications. Oblique views of vertebral arteries (Fig. 3-4) commonly disclose configurations and lumen sizes of origins and courses of proximal portions of these arteries, facts likely to be obscured in anteroposterior projections. Commonly vertebral arteries originate from the posterior aspect of subclavian arteries, and pathology and pathway can be appreciated best, if not solely, in oblique projecting angiograms. Such information has contributed to concepts helpful in devising improved operative procedures required to relieve pathophysiologic processes. Limited operative exposure is possible when precise location and extent of diseased arteries are demonstrated completely by three-dimensional angiograms. Faintness of opacification, compared to density above and below a site, probably represent atheroma *en face,* which may be expected to be confirmed in profile or biplane views.

Lateral views usually give optimal delineation of carotid sinus and extracranial portion of internal carotid artery. The normal carotid sinus has an enlarged diameter measuring 50 percent greater than that of the subsequent internal carotid artery.

Estimations of percent of stenoses consider normal sinus diameter as well as intrusions upon it. Ulcerated plaques occasionally are diagnosed by profile irregularity, by crater not dissimilar to the characteristic ulcer seen in gastrointestinal x-rays, and by contrasting densities.

Total versus near-total occlusion of internal carotid artery has different significances regarding flow and potential for reconstruction. Stenosis of internal carotid artery may be so pronounced that flow is delayed, and contrast medium may arrive late and diluted. Nearly all the flow into the common carotid artery may issue through the external carotid artery, and observers may overlook a strand of contrast in the internal carotid artery. Single exposures and faulty processing contribute to this oversight. Adequate technical angiograms provide indirect evidence of patency of the intraosseous course of the internal carotid artery, demonstrated as filling of the siphon via ophthalmic artery collateral circulation. This inference of patency beyond the straight, accessible extracranial segment of internal carotid artery is important in decisions to operate upon patients, and such interpretations and actions affect statistics. Twenty-five to 40 percent of occluded internal carotid arteries have been reported to have been reopened by endarterectomy, and a majority of these remained open, witnessed by

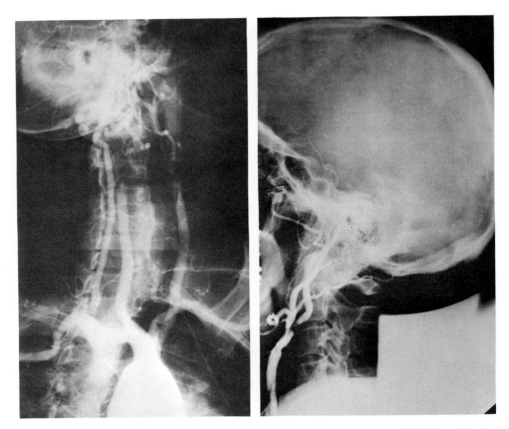

Figure 3-2 (left). DEFICIENCIES OF ARCH AORTOGRAPHY. This best-of-series arch angiogram lacks the advantages of selective studies. Despite exaggerated contrast of arch of aorta, there is inadequate detail of origins of vertebral arteries and course and structure of left vertebral artery. There is insufficient information concerning carotid bifurcations to form an opinion of operability.

The principle of angiography is the provision of precise anatomic information to enable specific diagnosis. Contemplation of corrective surgical operation demands intra- and extracranial functional (flow patterns) and structural information.

Figure 3-3 (right). CAROTID ARTERY STENOSIS. Lateral projection angiogram commonly best shows stenoses of internal carotid artery near origin. Three mechanisms can explain this near-total occlusion: (1) accumulation of lipids which comprise usual atheroma; (2) thrombus superimposed upon irregular plaque, abetted by slow flow; and (3) intramural hematoma, compressing lumen as intima yields to greater degree than adventitia. There is evidence of iatrogenic intramural abnormality of common carotid artery near needle site. The protrusion defect immediately proximal to the stenosis is consistent with an ulcerated plaque. The ulceration (not infrequently) may have eroded the lining, allowing evacuation of semisolid material, replaced by blood; dissection, hematoma, thrombosis follow. This may be one mechanism of acute occlusion. (See also Fig. 4-19.)

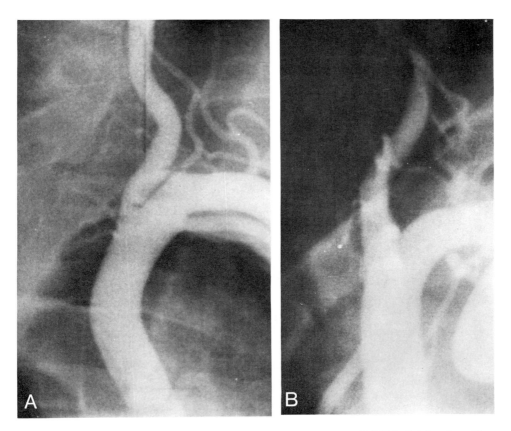

Figure 3-4. SYMPTOMATIC VERTEBRAL ARTERY STENOSIS. LAO view illustrates high-grade stenosis, elongation, and poststenotic dilatation. Lesion and symptoms were relieved by operation.

angiography at intervals after operation. The authors' experience is that operation can reestablish flow through the internal carotid artery if occlusion had not existed (misinterpretation or inadequacy of angiogram), if there was retrograde filling of the siphon, or if the occlusion was recent. Reopening has been accomplished rarely in the absence of these conditions. Improved balloon catheters have aided removal of thrombus distal to arteriotomy site.

Disruption of continuity of intima (ulceration) may occur with minimal or marked stenoses. The silhouette of the contrast medium lies contiguous with but projects from the stream of opaque substance. Not all ulcerated lesions seen at operation or autopsy are visible on angiograms, even though they may have been taken shortly before the plaque was observed. Ulcerations appear to have increased importance clinically, and their detection radiographically is not difficult in the typical case. Ulcerations at the carotid bifurcation and in the proximal portion of the internal carotid artery appear to be more common than those appearing in the intraosseous portion (Fig. 3-5). Stenoses of the intraosseous and cavernous

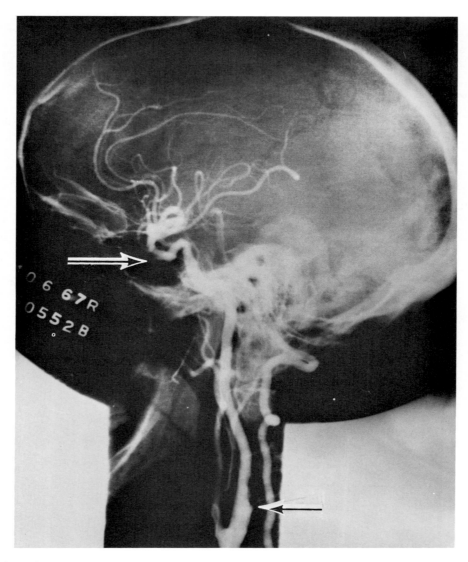

Figure 3-5. ULCERATED PLAQUES. These are evident at extracranial and intracranial locations of internal carotid artery.

portions of the internal carotid artery are common. A combination of lesions at the carotid bifurcation and intracranially are referred to as tandem lesions, each contributing to diminished flow and pressure. Stenosing or occluding lesions within the subdivisions of the internal carotid artery are of great clinical significance, but currently are beyond the reach of usual surgical therapeutic measures. Interesting confirmation of the sequence of events in the history may be reconstructed by attention to the locations of intracranial arterial stenoses.

CORONARY ANGIOGRAPHY

The safety of coronary angiography by experienced physicians prepared to treat ventricular arrhythmias has been established. Coronary angiography may be performed by supravalvular injection into the aorta, injections with catheter tip in an aortic sinus adjacent to right or left coronary arteries, and most precisely with intra-arterial passage of appropriate catheters. Specific projections outline individual arteries and their abnormalities to greatest advantage. Intra-arterial injection of antiadrengergic substances may disclose the ability of normal segments of arteries to change diameter, accentuating sites of atherosclerotic lesions of fixed diameter. Collateral patterns of circulation may be observed. Virtually total absence of circulation in some segments is consistent with fibrosis following infarction. Concurrent visualization of coronary arteries and ventricular cavity may confirm the presence or extent of ventricular aneurysm. Angiography during operation to evaluate reconstruction or bypass operations upon coronary arteries and indirect revascularization of myocardium by arterial implantation will be as important as the clinical state of the patient in estimating the virtues and short-comings of these procedures.

Indications for coronary angiography are relative. Patients with progressive or disabling angina may have obstructing processes in arteries with patent distal segments into which bypass grafts may be sutured. Normal electrocardiogram at rest may disclose abnormalities with exercise; these patterns in patients with progressive disabling ischemia suggest the advisability of coronary angiography. Mitral insufficiency following myocardial infarct may disable patients and require valve surgery. The contribution of revascularization of myocardium to prolonged survival seems reasonable, and long-term data is being accumulated.

A patient with a single episode of coronary occlusion without disabling angina is not a candidate for coronary artery surgery, and therefore visualization of the distribution and degree of coronary artery atherosclerotic processes is not warranted. Patients with minimal symptoms but several episodes of myocardial infarction may want to learn the possibility of precise treatment. Prognostic implications of coronary artery disease would appear to become better defined. Angiography and myocardial revascularization are not contraindicated by the presence of congestive heart failure, which is only a relative contraindication. Angiographic and surgical groups with favorable experience appear to be justified in studying the patient doomed by previous criteria of contraindications; congestive heart failure caused by aneurysm of the left ventricle is relieved by aneurysmectomy. Operative coronary angiography in two planes has yet to become common; doubtless it soon will. Myocardial scanning techniques may complement coronary angiography.

CELIAC AND MESENTERIC ANGIOGRAPHY

Technical difficulties of celiac and mesenteric angiography have been surmounted, and diagnostic accuracy is increasing with experience. Anatomic variations may be disclosed by this method. The relation of such anomalies to functional pathology of the gastrointestinal tract has not been established.

Abdominal trauma generally is an indication of exploratory operation rather than angiography. Experience may further define the role of angiography in trauma. Atherosclerosis causes high grade stenoses of origins of celiac and mesenteric arteries in many patients who have few symptoms. Infrequently patients with gastrointestinal malfunction and weight loss may be found to have near total obstruction of both celiac and superior mesenteric arteries, or obstruction of one and high grade stenosis of the second. Large bowel symptoms are not often caused by occlusion of the inferior mesenteric artery; the latter is common with abdominal aortic aneurysm without specific gastrointestinal symptoms. Emboli with occlusion of the superior mesenteric artery originating in the heart or aorta causes sudden severe typical symptoms of ischemia, leading to early operation rather than angiography. The high death rate from delayed diagnosis suggests that many aged people with vague abdominal symptoms might be salvaged if such symptoms led to early use of abdominal (celiac-mesenteric) angiography. Early postoperative angiography may be indicated in patients in whom resections of intestine have been required. One alternative has been the second look operation 24 hours after the first procedure. Experience may disclose that angiography has important contributions to make in patients who develop unsuspected ischemia after abdominal operations, and angiography may preclude the unnecessary second look operations in specific instances. Many tumors of the pancreas and some of the liver and gastrointestinal tract are precisely diagnosed by celiac or mesenteric angiography.

RENAL ANGIOGRAPHY

Survey angiography of renal arteries, in conjunction with visualization of the aorta and its branches to the lower extremities, can disclose unsuspected high grade stenoses, aneurysm, aberrant origin or multiple renal arteries, and occasionally cyst or tumor of the kidney. The search for a remediable cause of hypertension includes angiography. The presence of an epigastric bruit in a hypertensive patient would suggest the advisability of angiography as virtually the first step in hospital evaluation of the patient. Nonetheless, many such patients have prolonged hospitalizations and multiple indirect tests without the benefit of proof of normality or abnormality of the renal vasculature. This appears to represent errors of approach and judgment. Hypertension of recent origin unassociated with other stigmata of atherosclerosis and other known causes warrants renal angiography.

Suspected embolus to the kidney is a relative indication for angiography. Undeniably, early reprieve from ischemia is preferable to prolonged ischemia. Patients may be so ill from other causes (e.g., mitral stenosis with congestive heart failure and even pulmonary edema) that the renal complication of embolic arterial occlusion may seem of secondary importance. It may be equally important to know that the circulation to at least one kidney is intact as the basis for the clinical decision to permit the second kidney to suffer ischemic consequences, or for persisting with general systemic maintenance while the kidney with unobstructed circulation regains its function. Arterial hemorrhage may be the first indication of aneurysmal abnormality of the renal circulation and compression of renal veins from hematoma causing loss of renal function.

Renal failure may have intraluminal causes, or tubular function may have failed in the presence of intact major circulation. Stimulus to support vigorously a patient with intact circulation and transient tubular failure comes from knowledge that the circulation is intact. Injection of contrast medium may cause concern but it has not been proved that contrast media can cause irreparable damage to renal cells during acute tubular necrosis. Indeed, survival has occurred with subsequent near-normal renal function despite renal angiography superimposed upon prolonged periods of ischemia for arterial reconstruction.

Dicta carried over from contraindications to intravenous urography may not apply at all to arteriography. Commonly people with indications for renal arteriography have abnormalities of blood chemistry that are contraindications to IVP—elevated blood urea nitrogen and creatinine and diminished clearances of creatinine and test substances. Restored renal function may depend on improved vascularization which gets its greatest stimulus from angiographic demonstration that remediable (renovascular) causes are the bases of renal insufficiency.

AORTA ANGIOGRAPHY (AORTOGRAPHY)

All segments of the aorta have been resected with survival and function of patients. The entire aorta from origin to bifurcation has not been replaced in a single individual to date.

CONGENITAL MALFORMATIONS.   Aplasia, stenosis, coarctation, aneurysm, and fistulas at various sites of the thoracic and abdominal aorta may threaten the life or function of the patient or of specific organs; precise definition of lesions influencing clinical judgment may be obtained best by angiography. Aneurysms of the sinus of Valsalva are amenable to technical maneuvers. Fistulas from aortic sinuses to cardiac chambers may be localized by angiography and treated surgically. Windows between aorta and pulmonary artery in the ascending or descending (ductus) portions may be localized by cardiac catheterization in conjunction with selective angiography. Abnormal origins of coronary arteries from the pulmonary artery, abnormal origins and courses of pulmonary arteries from the ascending aorta (truncus arteriosus), or aberrant subclavian arteries may be diagnosed and the potential indications for operative correction assessed. Aberrant origins of great vessels to the upper extremities and brain or obliteration of them may be diagnosed by regional angiography. Aplasia of the proximal portion of the descending aorta is uncommon. Angiography is instrumental in the diagnosis of coarctations of preductal, postductal, or abdominal aortas, aberrant or multiple branches of visceral arteries, arteriovenous communications in retroperitoneal areas, and pelvic kidney arterial supply. Marfan's syndrome leads to degenerative process in early and midadult life causing aneurysms of the ascending aorta. Aneurysms of intercostal arteries may be associated with coarctation of the aorta and may be unsuspected except by demonstration with angiography.

ACQUIRED MALFORMATIONS. *Infections.* Mycotic aneurysms may occur from bacteremias or secondary to lodging of infected emboli in vessels. Infection at sites of arterial surgery (interruption of patent ductus arteriosus, resection of coarctation of aorta) may lead to aneurysm formation. Syphilitic aneurysms have been rare in the past decade. Characteristically they were fusiform involving the descending thoracic aorta. Untreated, even in patients in middle age, their erosion of vertebrae and sternum was seen and was symptomatic.

Trauma. Laceration of the thoracic aorta distal to the left subclavian artery can occur by abrupt interruption of forward motion as in auto accidents with steering wheel injury of the chest. Similarly, fistulas from aortic sinuses into cardiac chambers in some instances have been noted only after blunt trauma to the chest.

Degeneration. Dissecting aneurysm of the aorta has been classified as: Type 1—extending from the ascending aorta to various distances into the distal aorta (10 percent); Type 2—near the aortic annulus (9 percent); Type 3—originating distal to the left subclavian artery (81 percent).

Many variations of pathologic anatomy and functional consequences occur. There may be reentry of the false lumen at sites within the thoracic aorta or extending into iliac arteries. Rupture into pericardium, pleural space, or retroperitoneum may occur. Arteries may be sheared completely from the aorta with exsanguinating sequelae. Indications for angiography are strong clinical history, ischemia of vital part, expanding size, and threatened rupture. In the absence of progressive symptoms and signs, some surgeons advocate demonstration of communication between two lumina as the indication for surgical treatment. With such criteria angiography appears indicated in every instance of dissecting aneurysm to determine criteria for operation. Some physicians advocate nonoperative therapy in patients without progressive symptoms and signs, and angiography has nothing to offer in this set of circumstances.

Aneurysms of any portion of the thoracic aorta may occur as a consequence of atherosclerosis, but they are much more common in the infrarenal portion of the abdominal aorta. Some physicians believe that the origin of the lesion from an infrarenal location is virtually assured in every instance, and abdominal aortography is not indicated. However, there are many reasons why we employ angiography routinely before aneurysmectomy. Remediable disease of renal arteries may be disclosed. Finding aneurysmal abnormalities of the aorta at the site of renal arteries and proximally increases the risk of operation and is considered by some a contraindication to attempted operation.

At the distal extent of the usual aneurysm, remediable vascular disease frequently is diagnosed by angiography and permits the surgeon to improve the circulation to the extremities as a dividend to excision of the aneurysm. Unsuspected aneurysm with intraluminal thrombus may be disclosed when Seldinger catheter technique of retrograde passage of a catheter demonstrates the catheter outside the channel of contrast medium. Arterio-arterial emboli are more common in patients with aneurysm and ulcerated aortic abnormalities. Statistics have shown a low incidence of rupture of aneurysms less than 6 cm in diameter in the abdominal aorta and a five-year survival rate in nonoperated subjects with such aneurysms in excess of 30 percent in consecutive series over long periods in certain hospitals. It is to be remembered, however, that this is well below the five-year survival rate, including the operative mortality of 50 percent in consecutive series of patients of comparable ages whose aneurysms were treated by surgical operation.

Renal insufficiency is not an absolute contraindication to renal angiography. Angiography may disclose an abnormality with the implication that only the surgical treatment of that abnormality would permit prolongation of life. Postoperative angiograms disclose faults of materials and techniques which encourage their immediate replacement or correction rather than anticipating and explaining complications (Fig. 3-6).

ILIAC ANGIOGRAPHY

The absence of femoral pulses indicates obstruction at a higher level. The presence of palpable pulses in the infrarenal aorta localizes the obstruction within the iliac artery. Iliac artery obstructions may be secondary to marked kinking in association with large abdominal aortic aneurysm, to thrombus superimposed upon an atherosclerotic lesion, or to embolus. Good nutrition of an extremity, despite the absence of iliac pulses, implies patent profunda femoris artery or superficial femoral artery and distal arteries. Thus, localization of correctable pathology may not be difficult, but the precise mapping of normal or abnormal sites proximally and distally can be very useful in planning an operation. The likelihood of finding multiple, correctable lesions on the same or both sides and possibly in the abdominal aorta, are indications to strongly consider angiography although its use is not absolutely essential.

Iliac angiography may be useful even though a male patient may not have symptoms of vascular insufficiency of hypogastric arteries and their branches. Commonly, the atherosclerotic process is so extensive in the external iliac artery that angiographic visualization can warn the surgeon of pitfalls of attempted operation without providing for long-term continuity of the lumen of the iliac artery by bypass graft or direct arterial procedure. The proximal two centimeters of the external iliac artery have been found to be markedly stenotic in many patients in whom aorto-iliac obstruction (Leriche syndrome) is found. Such abnormalities may be demonstrated on preoperative angiograms and remain uncorrected in postoperative angiograms. Preoperative angiography permits estimation of the magnitude of operation and the prognosis, and in turn can influence decisions regarding operation. Assessment of quantity and pressure of flow through aorta and iliac segments influences long-term patency of peripheral arterial reconstructive surgery. Accordingly, all patients in whom reconstructive operations of the periphery are planned stand to benefit from preoperative visualization of aorta, iliac, femoral, popliteal, and distal arteries.

Acute ischemia of the periphery in the absence of palpable infrarenal aortic pulse indicates the need for immediate operative relief of obstruction of the distal aorta and proximal iliac arteries. Plans should be made for intraopera-

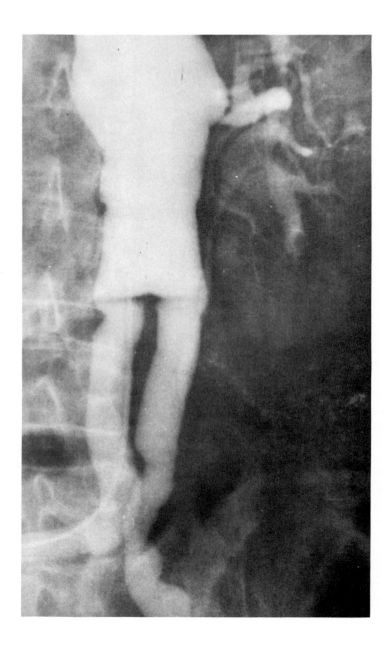

Figure 3-6. ROUTINE POSTOPERATIVE ANGIOGRAPHY. Kinked origins of bifurcation graft; the limbs are too long. The bifurcation of the graft is appropriately high, at L3. (Scarcely visible is the bypass graft from left common iliac to left renal artery, due to this film early in the series.) Previous right nephrectomy for contracted kidney and hypertension. This obese, markedly hypertensive, uremic septuagenarian died 5 years later of ruptured aorta proximal to renal arteries.

tive flow studies and angiography after removal of the major obstructing mechanism. It is permissible to avoid the delay of preoperative angiography outside the operating suite. There is neither debate nor delay in hospitals where physician and radiologist are psychologically prepared to provide all diagnostic services as promptly as required by the urgency of the circumstances. A relative contraindication emphasizes the need for thoughtful planning and implementation of a procedure rather than banning it. For example, in instances of aortic and iliac artery obstruction, deposit of contrast medium above the site of obstruction will obligate much flow into visceral and spinal arteries with greater potential for damage from excess doses or increased concentrations. Small quantities of contrast medium appropriately placed proximal to the aortic obstruction can be useful without threatening damage.

FEMORAL ANGIOGRAPHY

Angiograms may disclose arteriovenous aneurysms localized between the groin and ankle, which are treatable if localized to one or a few specific sites. Laceration or division of arteries with or without arteriovenous communication may be demonstrated following blunt or sharp trauma. Delineation of circulation distal to femoral or popliteal arteries can be most helpful in planning operative procedures. Thrombosis in an aneurysm or proximal or distal to it may indicate the need for a bypass graft. Patency of arteries on either side of an aneurysm suggests the feasibility of excision and restoration of continuity by graft if necessary. Emboli are a special indication for angiography. Multiple emboli may not be suspected when a large embolus is present in a classical site (Fig. 3-7). The distinction between embolus and thrombosis may be suggested when coexistent atherosclerosis is seen, indicating the need to be prepared for arterial reconstructive surgery in addition to embolectomy. Angiography must precede amputation in most instances of ischemia secondary to trauma, atherosclerosis, or diabetes mellitus.

There are a few contraindications to visualization of the femoral arteries. The technique of the procedure may vary, depending upon local anatomic conditions, hospital facilities, and experience of the operator. Specifically, infection in the foot, cellulitis, and lymphangitis below the knee do *not* contraindicate percutaneous femoral angiography. Massive edema, inflammation, and lymphagitis at the groin may suggest the advisability of translumbar or axillary routes. Rarely is the common femoral artery inaccessible to skilful percutaneous placement of a needle even in the absence of pulsations. At times the lumen in the common femoral artery is small, and an 18-gauge Cournand needle will enter the artery, whereas a larger cannula generally used for insertion of guide wire and catheter is too large. At times inability to enter an artery is a matter of ill fortune; uncommonly, it is due to total absence of lumen. In the latter instance placement of the needle slightly more distally will permit entering the bifurcation of the common femoral artery or the profunda femoris artery. If the limb is viable the proximal portions of the profunda femoris artery almost certainly must be patent.

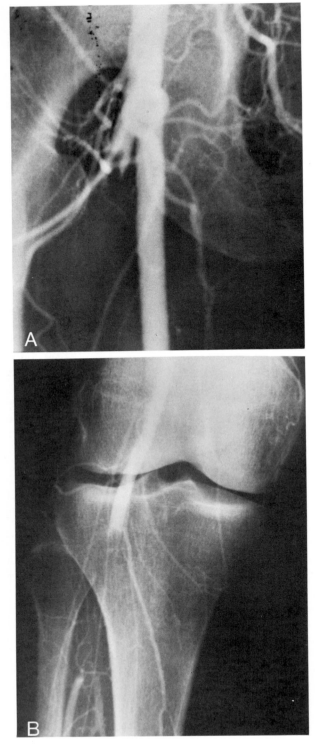

Figure 3-7. ROUTINE ANGIOGRAPHY DISCOVERS ALL EMBOLI

It is most desirable to have all possible information available prior to operation. The certainty of entering the lumen of a vessel that has been exposed by surgical operation may be greater than percutaneous puncture in some hands, but there are important shortcomings to "cutdown arteriography"—time involved, less satisfactory angiographic equipment in an operating room, and exposure of a wound to contamination at a time remote from a surgical procedure. Femoral angiography is indicated after embolectomy if all peripheral pulses have not been restored. This should be a routine procedure in the operating room. Blind distal passage of balloon catheters for embolectomy is not a recommended procedure (see p. 77); however, in instances where it is used, the importance of angiography before and after such blind maneuvers will emphasize their needlessness and the virtue or the harm of such procedures by surgeons who do practice such maneuvers routinely.

Angiography is to be performed following in-situ vein bypass graft operations (Fig. 3-8) and virtually any kind of arterial reconstruction distal to the femoral triangle. Again, the quality and virtue of serial angiograms may make it more advisable to defer the procedure till the postoperative period. In these instances, angiograms within a day or two of operation, with introduction of the needle above the operative site, can disclose abnormalities threatening thrombosis before it occurs (Fig. 3-9). Thus, early discovery of the need for a remediable procedure occurs soon enough to minimize delay. A smaller volume and greater density of contrast medium may be directed into the vessels regionally by injection through a femoral needle rather than through a catheter placed at a higher level.

Occlusive processes of the distal femoral, entire popliteal, and proximal tibial and peroneal arteries may make conventional reconstruction difficult or impossible. Here it is even more important that adequate angiograms of the distal arteries be obtained (Fig. 3-10). The criteria of inoperability of a few years ago have changed, and long bypass operations to distal vessels of the leg, ankle, and foot are now virtually routine and highly successful. They are such an acceptable substitute to ablation of limbs that the angiographer must provide the patient with every opportunity for salvage of the limb. Techniques to improve the quality of visualization include injection of larger quantities of contrast medium over a longer period of time with serial films taken for extended periods. Measures to increase the diameter of vessels include reactive hyperemia, intra-arterial injection of 30 mg papaverine, or second injection of contrast medium soon after the first. It has been observed that spasm which may be apparent with an injection of contrast medium may be followed by relaxation of that spasm which does not recur with a second injection.

Figure 3-7. Emboli in profunda femoris and in popliteal arteries in the same patient. (A) The former can elude detection by physical examination. (B) Embolic occlusion of distal popliteal artery obstructs origins of anterior tibial artery and tibioperoneal trunk.

The correct operation for emboli at this location is local operative exposure of anterior and posterior tibial and peroneal arteries, to assure entry of Fogarty catheter into posterior tibial, peroneal, anterior tibial, and proximal popliteal arteries, in that order.

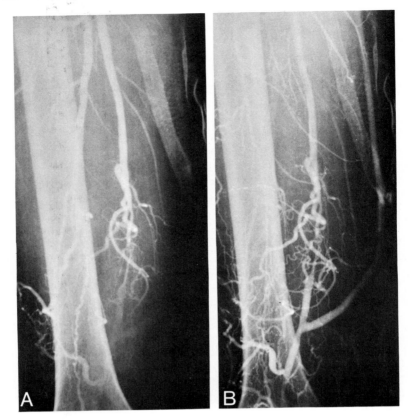

Figure 3-8. POPLITEAL-SAPHENOUS "STEAL" VIA IN-SITU GRAFT. (A) Early phase of injection of superficial (occluded) and deep femoral arteries. (B) Later in sequence, contrast medium is ascending the in-situ graft, while the popliteal artery is scarcely visualized.

Angiography by injection of contrast medium into popliteal and tibial arteries is a procedure that requires operative exposure. It is generally done in the operating room in conjunction with exploration or with attempted reconstruction. It is permissible as a substitute for amputation; however, exploration of popliteal and distal arteries is rarely an acceptable substitute for properly performed serial angiography.

BLOOD FLOW MEASUREMENTS

Blood flow describes passage through conduit vessels (arteries), capacitance vessels (veins), and arteriovenous shunts. Noncannulating electromagnetic flow probes readily supply these data at operation. Radioactive macroaggregates afford similar data. Perfusion is the term used to denote circulation through exchange (nutritive) vessels, the capillaries. Muscle and skin circulation are examples of vascular beds in which perfusion is measured by plethysmography.

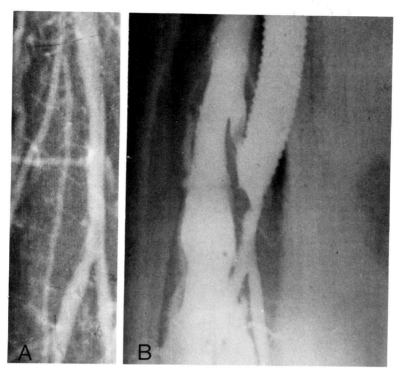

Figure 3-9. CLAMP TRAUMA. (A) Angiogram of tibioperoneal artery. (B) Trauma of vascular clamps caused filling defects immediately proximal to site of anastomosis of cloth graft to artery, and near bifurcation of tibioperoneal artery. (The prominent venous filling is secondary to an arteriovenous fistula created distally).

Effective blood flow to the periphery and perfusion to end organs are basic to normal function. Physical examination permits clinical estimation of relative normalcy and adequacy of flow (pulses), and perfusion as judged by appearance, temperature, and venous filling time. Angiography records patency and transit time of contrast media, and radiologists use these criteria in defining normal and abnormal and adequate and inadequate blood flow. Absolute values and relative changes in flow, perfusion, and angiograms are used to describe physical and physiologic status and to define responses to heat, exercise, drug infusion, changed viscosity, and surgical reconstruction.

The lowest incidence of failure of maintained patency weeks to months after operation requires more than satisfaction with appearance of the limb, graft, angiogram, or technical details of procedure. These alone do not assure a surgeon a palpable pulse in the segment beyond the distal arteriotomy site. While it is a useful practice to include distal sites of palpation of pulses in the sterile operative field to permit this clinical evaluation, angiography, flow studies, and responses to vasoactive drugs contribute more to the objective evaluation. The volume of

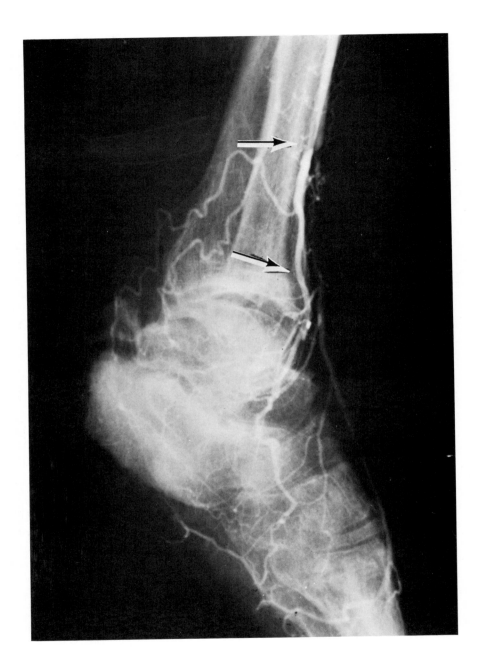

Figure 3-10. BIPLANE SERIAL ANGIOGRAPHY. Discontinuity of anterior tibial artery 3 inches above ankle joint. Peroneal artery branches conducted contrast material into a branch of anterior tibial artery, from which dorsalis pedis artery was visualized (AP view alone failed to illustrate discontinuity and overlap).

blood flowing to calf muscles and to the foot as a consequence of femoropopliteal artery reconstruction is the information which best describes adequacy of technical results and probability of long-term patency. The Whitney mercury-in-silastic plethysmographic strain gauge is readily gas sterilized and has been found useful in the operating room in supplying highly reproducible measurements of blood flow to calf muscles distal to common sites of termination of arterial reconstruction below or above the knee.

Since plethysmography and radioactive techniques are not used by most surgeons, but electromagnetic flow probes are used by many, placement of the probe beyond the distal anastomosis is likely to provide the most meaningful data. The common practice of applying the flow probe to the common femoral artery for ease of application and for ready comparison with measurements made at that site prior to arterial reconstruction must be modified. Observed increases in flow in the common femoral artery may be accurate, but they are secondary to reactive hyperemia or to flow into the huge muscle mass of the thigh. To determine distal flow without masking imperfections in reconstruction that may limit flow beyond the distal site of anastomosis or reconstruction, there must be transient occlusion of major branches of the artery to which the probe is applied.

Broad ranges of "normal" flow measured with noncannulating electromagnetic flow meters have been published. Greater than 50 percent increases in flow following intra-arterial injection of papaverine (30 mg) have been equated with patent distal bed (adequate run-off). Failure to increase flow with papaverine suggests technical error or limited flow potential (inadequate run-off).

Following aorta-femoral bypass grafts, patients exhibit 250 to 500 ml/min average flow through the common femoral artery. Bernhard, Ellison, and colleagues[3] recorded 270 ml/min, and Golding and Cannon[7] cited 550 ml/min. Bernhard's lowest flow rate at this site with maintained patency was 60 ml/min.

In eleven patients in both Golding's and Bernhard's series, blood flow through femoral-popliteal bypass grafts averaged 130 ml/min. Our data is similar, and papaverine usually increases flow 50 to 100 percent. Creation of arteriovenous fistula distal to such grafts tripled the flow. Mannick[13] reported lowest flow rate consistent with prolonged patency of femoral-popliteal bypass graft as 30 ml/min, and Bernhard's[3] observation cited flow rates as low as 15 ml/min consistent with patency for many months.

Average total cerebral blood flow in normal subjects is 1100 ml/min in women and 1300 ml/min in men. Kety and Schmidt[10] find it reasonable to apportion half of this unilaterally (± 600 ml/min), with perhaps two-thirds (400 ml) to carotid and one-third (200 ml) to vertebral artery distribution. Golding and Cannon[7] reported blood flow studies in carotid arteries of ten patients, in whom average flow in internal carotid arteries was 68 ml/min before surgical relief of stenosis, and 149 ml/min subsequently. Our figures were 83 and 206, respectively.

All these figures may hide more than they disclose unless explanation is provided for discrepancies from expected results. Indices of cardiac output, response to drugs, gas tensions, and altered viscosity and angiography would permit more precise evaluation of the blood flow data.

It is alleged that errors of interpretation underlie certain reports of increased blood flow following sympathectomy. Blood flow recorded in common femoral artery before, immediately after, and at intervals of several months following lumbar sympathectomy in different patients casts no light on the essential goal (regional perfusion distally). The reported increases in flow at all intervals, early and late, cited as evidences that sympathectomy does increase blood flow in the femoral artery, does not answer the important question: Was blood flow increased, and maintained, in the sites requiring it?

Observation reported by Redisch, Tangco, and Saunders[19] indicated decreased muscle flow early and late after resection of lumbar ganglia 1 to 4. Failure to sustain even the early increases of flow to skin was noted with passage of time. In contrast to expected responses following sympathectomy skin and muscle circulation decreased in response to body warming. Exercise decreased skin perfusion. Norepinephrine elicited greater constrictor response in skin than it did when the sympathetic nervous system was intact.

BIBLIOGRAPHY

1. ANSON, B. J., RICHARDSON, G. A., and MINEAR, W. L. Variations in number and arrangement of renal vessels: A study of blood supply of 400 kidneys. *J. Urol.*, 36:211, 1936.

2. BERANBAUM, S. L., and MEYERS, P. H., eds. *Special Procedures in Roentgen Diagnosis.* Springfield, Ill., Charles C Thomas, Publisher, 1963.

3. BERNHARD, V. M., KAYSER, K., GUTIENEZ, J. E., WILSON, S. D., RODGERS, R. E., and ELLISON, E. H. Salvage of ischemic limb. *J.A.M.A.*, 204:234, 1968.

4. DASELER, E. H., and ANSON, B. J. Surgical anatomy of the subclavian artery and its branches. *Surg. Gynec. Obstet.*, 108:149, 1959.

5. DAVIS, E., and LANDAU, J. *Clinical Capillary Microscopy.* Springfield, Ill., Charles C Thomas, Publisher, 1966.

6. GIBBON, J. H., and LANDIS, E. M. Vasodilation in the lower extremities in response to immersing the forearm in warm water. *J. Clin. Invest.*, 11:5, 1932.

7. GOLDING, A. L., and CANNON, J. A. Application of electromagnetic blood flowmeter during arterial reconstruction: Results in conjunction with papaverine in 47 cases. *Ann. Surg.*, 164:662, 1966.

8. HASS, W. K., FIELDS, W. S., NORTH, R. R., KRICHEFF, I. I., CHASE, N. E., and BAUER, R. B. Joint study of extracranial arterial occlusion. II: Arteriography, techniques, sites, and complications. *J.A.M.A.*, 203:961, 1968.

9. INGVAR, D. H., and LASSEN, N. A. *Regional cerebral blood flow. Acta Neurol. Scand.*, Suppl. 14, 1965.

10. KETY, S. S., and SCHMIDT, C. F. The effects of altered arterial tensions of carbon dioxide and oxygen on cerebral blood flow and cerebral oxygen consumption of normal young men. *J. Clin. Invest.*, 27:484, 1948.

11. LASSEN, N. A. Muscle blood flow in normal man and in patients with intermittent claudication evaluated by simultaneous Xe^{133} and Na^{24} clearance. *J. Clin. Invest.*, 43:1805, 1964.

12. LAUFMAN, H., BERGGREN, R. E., FINLEY, T., and ANSON, B. J. Anatomical studies of the lumbar arteries, with reference to the safety of translumbar aortography. *Ann. Surg.*, 152:621, 1960.

13. MANNICK, J. A., and JACKSON, B. T. Hemodynamics of arterial surgery in atherosclerotic limbs. I. Direct Measurement of blood flow before and after vein grafts. *Surgery*, 59:713, 1966.

14. McCormack, L. J., Cauldwell, E. W., and Anson, B. J. Brachial and antebrachial arterial patterns: A study of 750 extremities. *Surg. Gynec. Obstet.*, 96:43, 1953.

15. Michels, N. A. *Blood Supply and Anatomy of the Upper Abdominal Organs.* Philadelphia, J. B. Lippincott Co., 1955.

16. Mueller, O. *Die Kapillaren der menschlichen Koerperoberflaeche in gesunden und kranken Tagen.* Stutigart, Enke, 1922.

17. Muller, R. F., and Figley, M. M. The arteries of the abdomen, pelvis, and thigh. I. Normal roentgenographic anatomy; II. Collateral circulation in obstructive arterial disease. *Amer. J. Roentgen.*, 77:296, 1957.

18. Nyboer, J. *Electrical Impedance Plethysmography.* Springfield, Ill., Charles C Thomas, Publisher, 1970.

19. Redisch, W., Tangco, F. F., and Saunders, R. L. *Peripheral Circulation in Health and Disease.* New York, Grune & Stratton, Inc., 1957.

20. Strandness, D. E., Jr. *Peripheral Arterial Diseases.* Boston, Little, Brown and Company, 1969.

20. Winsor, T., and Hyman, C. *A Primer of Peripheral Vascular Diseases.* Philadelphia, Lea Febiger, 1965.

22. Wood, J. E. *The Veins.* Boston, Little Brown and Company, 1965.

CHAPTER 4

RESTORATION OF PRIMARY CIRCULATION

INDICATIONS

Arteries may be operated upon when there is a remediable obstructive process causing serious symptoms or threatening incapacity. Circulatory deficiency may interfere with gainful employment or enjoyment of living; it may cause pain with effort or at rest or threaten loss of function or viability of tissue. Arteries must be susceptible to long-term patency after reconstruction by at least one of the available techniques. Patients must be well enough to survive operation and to benefit from the required corrective procedure.

CONTRAINDICATIONS

Contraindications to attempts to restore mainline circulation are relative. The physician may estimate the probable systemic and local consequences of inadequate circulation without restoration by operation. The experience of the vascular surgeon permits estimation of operability by angiography and prediction of results. There is a spectrum of pathologic states in arteries, some so favorable that technical success is virtually assured, others so extensive that neither early nor long-term patency can be anticipated with certainty. Physician and patient may elect an attempt at salvage rather than accept certain amputation.

PROCEDURES IN ATHEROSCLEROSIS

Atherosclerosis produces focal and diffuse lesions, and both may cause significant impediments to volume and rate of blood flow, especially when they occur in sequence. Treatment of each is possible, the effects enhancing comfort, enjoyment, and productivity of the lives of many patients. Indications for reconstruction may be elective to relieve discomfort, disability, or threat of thrombosis, or it may be absolute, the alternative being death of the part or of the patient. Contraindications to any operation and to specific procedures do exist; patients may be too ill with associated diseases, or the ischemic part may be beyond salvage. Technical considerations may preclude successful outcome. It is well to remember that the mortality rate in patients with above-knee amputation exceeds 25 percent, and the rate of nonhealing of below-knee amputations exceeds 25 percent.

THROMBOENDARTERECTOMY

Thromboendarterectomy yields satisfactory results when the procedure is performed carefully with strict attention to technical details. Successful reestablishment of circulation may be anticipated when the distal peripheral vessels are patent and there is an adequate run-off space. The important goal is the restoration of pulsatile blood flow into the peripheral arterial tree. The selection of endarterectomy indicates that one expects from it as satisfactory a result as from any of the procedures available, plus some additional advantages. It is clear that appropriate matching of procedure with lesion influences results of operation. The least technical difficulty achieving optimal result is anticipated when a short stenotic lesion is totally removed from a vessel of large caliber.

Angiography is paramount in selection of patients for surgery. A spectrum of lesions appears which affects results of surgical treatment. Angiograms may disclose obliterative disease that is totally unremediable by direct operative approach. In some patients, one may infer little likelihood of success and in others, small chance of failure. Angiography is used to identify the nature and extent of pathology. Contrast substances must be seen in vessels proximal and distal to the intended operative site. Inferring the presence or distribution of contrast medium, rather than seeing it and the pathology that must be demonstrated, is a major error of the inexperienced physician.

Endarterectomy is intended to open orifices of numerous collateral branches as well as segments of the main channel. The *atherosclerotic process* affects surgical outcome. Frequently atheromata are firm and fibrous or calcified (mature) and lend themselves to removal; such lesions fall out by themselves. However, atheromata may be nonuniform in penetration and adherence to vessel wall at different sites, at bifurcation, in orifices, and for distances into branches. Here, the manipulations required and the incomplete removal and ragged bed that result may yield less favorable results.

The smoothness or roughness of *arterial lining* after endarterectomy is influenced in large measure by appropriate surgical technique. Arteriotomy and visualization of the entire atheromatous area should produce better results than indirect techniques. Strippers and spiral loops of wire, avulsing and abrading as they are forced through vessels may remove less obstructive material and create a thrombogenic vascular bed. Gas endarterectomy is alleged to yield smoother neointima.

MANAGEMENT OF INTIMA

Extensions of atheroma beyond orifices of collateral arteries are to be left undisturbed and in contact with underlying media. It is incorrect to grasp such plaques and avulse the presenting portion. Back-bleeding is not to be equated with likelihood of patency. The most important single technical step influencing patency of a vessel after endarterectomy is management of intima at the distal end of the arteriotomy. Bevelling of distal intima can be difficult. It is advisable to use a longitudinal arteriotomy incision carried beyond a plaque and terminated in a pliable vessel (Fig. 4-1). Intraluminal manipulation is to be terminated where visibility and technical management are optimal. Alternatively, transverse arteriotomy is made without elevating the distal atheroma. Actually, one still is managing the atheroma, with its qualities of friability and tendency to separate from media. Tacking sutures (Fig. 4-2) serve a limited purpose and thrombosis may be initiated near them. Rough surface and subintimal plane of dissection are both thrombogenic stimuli.

PRIMARY CLOSURE

Primary closure must leave an effective lumen size equal to proximal and distal vessels. If this has to be achieved by sutures taken too near the cut edge of the artery, wall strength may be sacrificed, and hematoma and disruption may occur. Whether primary closure or composite reconstruction is performed, constriction at the ends of the arteriotomy must be avoided. Sutures are not placed distal to the incision; they may be intended to anchor the continuous suture, but constriction results (Fig. 4-3). Sutures are placed one millimeter from ends of incisions and from edges of the arteriotomy. Separate sutures are used for each side of a patch; they are not started as mattress sutures, nor tied to each other. Excess diameter must be avoided when patches are used, to preclude ill effects of turbulent flow.

CLOSURE WITH PATCH GRAFT

Patches of vein or cloth may be necessary, but should not be used arbitrarily. A conduit of bigger bore is not a guarantee of patency. Optimal lumina of arteries are uniform in caliber. Over-sized patches (and it is difficult to avoid these) create turbulence; this leads to thrombosis.

Closing arteriotomies over catheters assures a given minimal lumen size, not necessarily uniform in caliber. *Each suture is placed as if it is the most important one.* Oiled 5-0 continuous silk suture is easy to use and has adequate strength. Polyethylene suture material is easy to work with and has advantages ascribed to monofilament sutures. Closure effected by placing sutures from atheroma to wall is less likely to initiate a false plane of dissection.

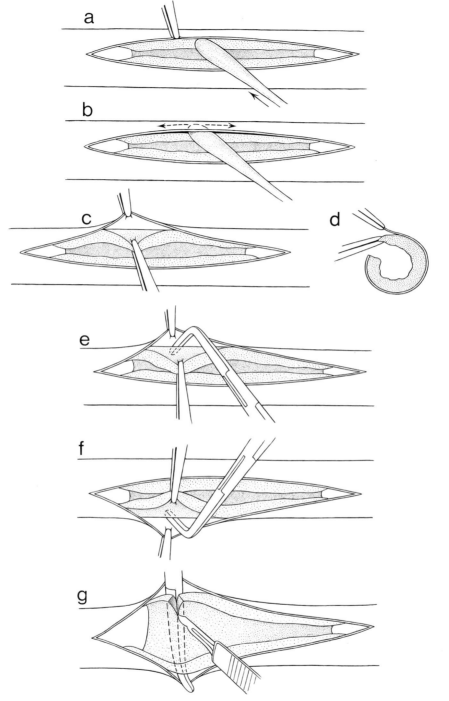

Figure 4-1. TECHNIQUE OF ENDARTERECTOMY. Incision is carried beyond limits of atheroma. Forceps grasps adventitia, and freer elevator seeks to initiate plane of dissection (a, b). Circumferential development of plane 180° from each side may be facilitated by curved clamp as forceps separate components (e, f). The bulk of atheroma is excised prior to precise tailoring of junction of residual atheroma with intima or with adventitia.

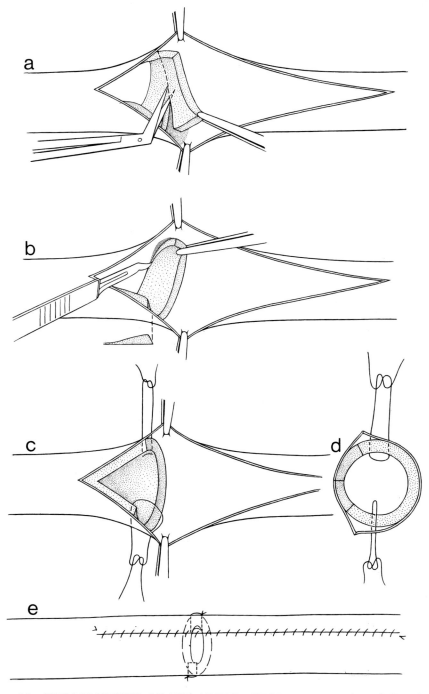

Figure 4-2. TERMINATION OF ENDARTERECTOMY. Irrespective of direction of flow, systolic pressure tends to overdistend endarterectomized segment. Thus, it is essential to excise plaque flush with media-adventitia (a, b), leaving neither thrombogenic surface nor leading point for intramural dissection. Minimal traction is applied to plaque, and even less to arterial wall, precluding need for tacking sutures. When used, tacking sutures may be placed transversely, both components inside-out on plaque (c, d, top), or longitudinally (c, d, bottom), when one or both limbs may penetrate plaque.

Figure 4-3. PRIMARY CLOSURE OF ARTERIOTOMY INCISION. All sutures bracket the arterial incision. (They do not show a common error of beginning beyond the arteriotomy site, in the intact artery, which results in constriction with loss of cross-sectional area.) Distances from incision and between sutures, and full-thickness penetration of walls assure that *each stitch is the most important one.* Traction upon each limb of the loop as the last suture is tied (c) permits adjustment of appropriate tension upon previously placed sutures. Correct tension approximates cut edges of artery; excess tension decreases caliber of host vessel (e).

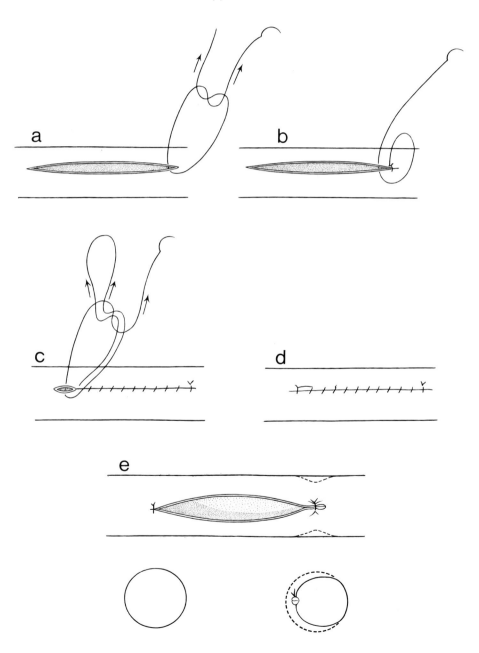

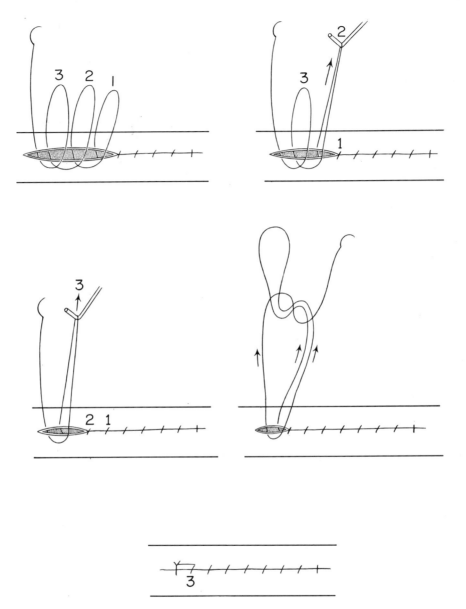

Figure 4-4. PRIMARY CLOSURE OF SMALL ARTERY. The last few sutures are placed without tension upon any, to preserve visibility for precise placement of each. The smaller the artery, the more important is every such detail.

Concepts and techniques successfully employed in aorta-iliac endarterectomy have been used at other sites. Using proximal and distal incisions, patency has been restored to narrowed orifices of the deep femoral, external carotid, vertebral, hypogastric, and visceral arteries. Attention to angiograms and correlation with symptoms may emphasize the need for the benefits of endarterectomy of these smaller branches. Longitudinal arteriotomy is placed 90 to 120 degrees away from the principal arteriotomy site. As in aorta-iliac endarterectomy, the lesser incision assures smooth arterial lining distally and aids removal of the stenosing lesions of the orifice. There appear to be special dividends in this extended operation upon profunda femoris artery orifices when obstruction of the distal aorta and iliac arteries is relieved and stenoses or occlusions of superficial femoral arteries coexist. Experience with angiography has demonstrated the relative paucity of symptoms in patients with obstructed superficial femoral arteries whose profunda femoris arteries are large and communicate readily with patent popliteal arteries through abundant collateral vessels. Approximately 50 percent of patients with these tandem lesions are relieved of claudication by revascularization of proximal arteries only. Enlarging the effective orifices of stenosed deep femoral arteries may contribute to this improved circulation. This procedure must be considered strongly when indicated by the angiogram and when the common femoral artery is entered as part of aorta-iliac reconstruction with the object of obviating femoro-popliteal reconstruction.

This operation is commended for its intrinsic value and as the advocated substitute for other less precise procedures. *Avulsing a plaque from the orifice of a vessel is condemned.* The technical limits of operability of small vessels are subjective and may be evaluated first by angiography, then by long-term patency (Fig. 4-4). Experience with deliberate technique (5-0 suture material, and magnifying loupe of 2.4× magnification and 10-inch focal length) permits vascular repair without stenoses of the second order branches of deep femoral and external carotid arteries (Figs. 4-5 and 4-6); plaques in these arteries are usually focal. By contrast, plaques in hypogastric arteries are extensive, exposure is limited, and record of patency is low when hypogastric artery branches are reconstructed.

PRESERVING ORIFICE SITES IN RECONSTRUCTION

The early techniques of vascular reimplantation of Carrel preserved a cuff of the parent artery, permitting placement of sutures at a distance from a tubular structure of critically small diameter where caliber and patency may be compromised by sutures in the small vessel. This technique offers advantages in anastomosing hypogastric and profunda femoris arteries to prosthetic grafts. These arteries may remain in situ, together with the dorsal wall of parent arteries. Onlay of a prosthetic graft may be done readily, creating a composite graft. Grafts of varying diameters may be joined at such sites with minimal transitional disproportion (Fig. 4-7).

BYPASS GRAFT

CORRECT HANDLING OF PLAQUES AND INSTRUMENTS

Fortunately, the most dense collection of sheet-like plaque usually is found on the dorsal wall of the aorta and iliac and common femoral arteries and recurs segmentally. This permits arteriotomy on the ventral (anterior or anteromedial)

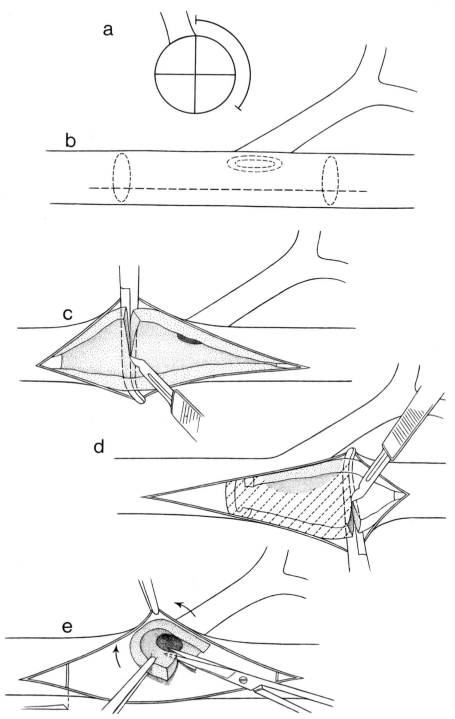

Figure 4-5. ENDARTERECTOMY OF ORIFICES AT BIFURCATIONS. Usual techniques of isolation and occlusion of arteries precede arteriotomy 120° from bifurcation. The plaque is dissected proximal (c) and distal (d) to the bifurcation, and the bulk (cross-hatched area) may be excised to permit visualization for precise excision of residual plaque (e) flush with origin of tributary. The plaque of the tributary is *never* avulsed.

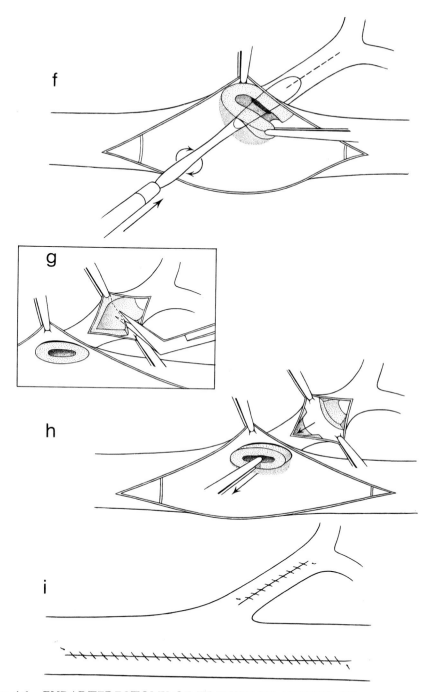

Figure 4-6. ENDARTERECTOMY OF TRIBUTARY ARTERY. When angiogram or inspection dictate endarterectomy into a tributary artery (carotid, femoral, renal), the bulk of that plaque is freed by maneuvers through the parent artery. A separate longitudinal incision insures precise termination and smooth transition onto lining of distal artery. Blind plucking of atheroma is decried, to preclude partial removal with fragmentation, residual plaque, thrombogenic surface, or intramural dissection and disruption.

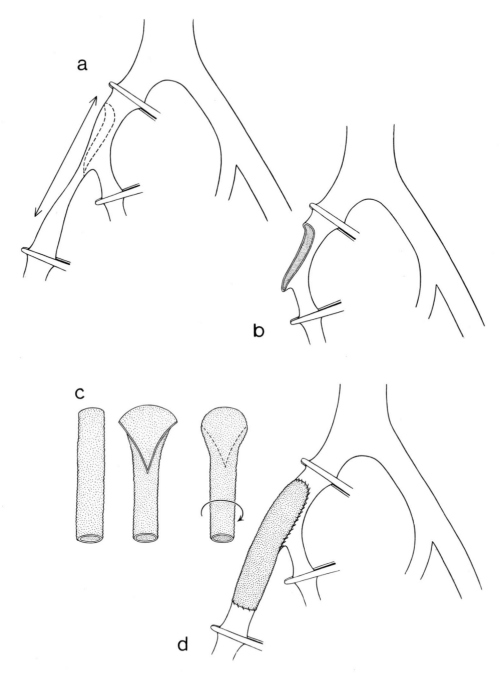

Figure 4-7. RECONSTRUCTION OF ORIFICES AT BIFURCATIONS. Stenoses of proximal portions of continuing major arterial trunks may occur primarily or subsequent to prior reconstruction. Prostheses, autografts or allografts may be fashioned as part onlay and part tubular conduits. (Note that clamps are portrayed as applying the more compressible anterior walls of arteries to the plate-like plaques that commonly are part of the dorsal walls of arteries.)

portion of the walls of arteries, at sites least involved with atheromata. Occluding clamps are best applied well away from the sites of arteriotomy, and loosely (i.e., to the first ratchet on the handle of the clamp), in a plane to compress the pliable wall against the rigid posterior wall (Fig. 4-8); this minimizes fragmentation (arterioarterial emboli) and separation of atheroma from the media (intramural dissection). Inspection of postoperative angiograms may disclose extensive trauma to atheromata inflicted by clamps (see Fig. 4-17, p. 79). However, this injurious effect is likely to be no more severe than that from application of circumferential tape compressed against tubing, or from application of broad blades of bulldog clamps. Multitooth clamps do not slip, and single application with appropriate compression produces trauma only once. Tension in the blades of clamps, length of teeth, and their geometric distribution affect relative occlusive forces or incisive consequences. Sharp-toothed clamps (Potts-Richter) were developed for application to pediatric vessels, whereas clamps with shorter teeth and diffuse configuration (DeBakey-Pilling) were developed for application to atherosclerotic vessels. Acceptable substitutes for clamping are insertion of catheters. Transient hemostasis is achieved by digital pressure as catheters are inserted. Alternatively, catheters may be inserted to assure restoration of caliber (if not surface integrity) as clamps are removed just prior to tying sutures already in place. When there is sufficient length of arteriotomy site, closed primarily or with a patch, clamps may be moved from the nonoperative site onto the reconstructed vessel which will not suffer from clamp trauma. However, the suture material may be weakened by clamping it.

Longitudinal incision started with a knife should penetrate all layers of one wall of the artery, to preclude separation of plaque from the wall and may be continued with knife or scissors. The practiced surgical hand can draw a blade longitudinally through adventitia and media into plaque substance and penetrate the full thickness of plaque. However, imprecise technique readily causes or permits separation of plaque from the pliable wall (permissible only during endarterectomy). Fine, sharp scissors whose action is cutting rather than crushing will open atheromatous arterial walls as a single layer and may be the preferred instrument after the initial penetration into the arterial lumen.

There is sufficient pliability in involved arterial walls to permit gaping of the arteriotomy site and maintenance of effective orifice size following graft implantation and restoration of blood flow. Usually it is neither required nor desirable to remove a button of tissue or to perform endarterectomy locally, for the end-result cannot provide as optimal a surface for blood flow as the non-traumatized vessel lining which is first encountered following expertly performed arteriotomy. An exception has been observed in the aorta, where linear incisions serving as orifice sites for vein grafts to coronary arteries have become sealed in a matter of months.. It does appear advisable to remove elliptical or circular segments of wall of the ascending aorta prior to suturing vein grafts to it. Occasionally, small vein grafts and their sites of implantation do require tailoring (Fig. 4-9).

There are several viewpoints concerning handling the arterial wall with forceps. A hands-off policy inflicts no trauma directly. However, precise and facile reconstruction demands visibility and control which may best be achieved with

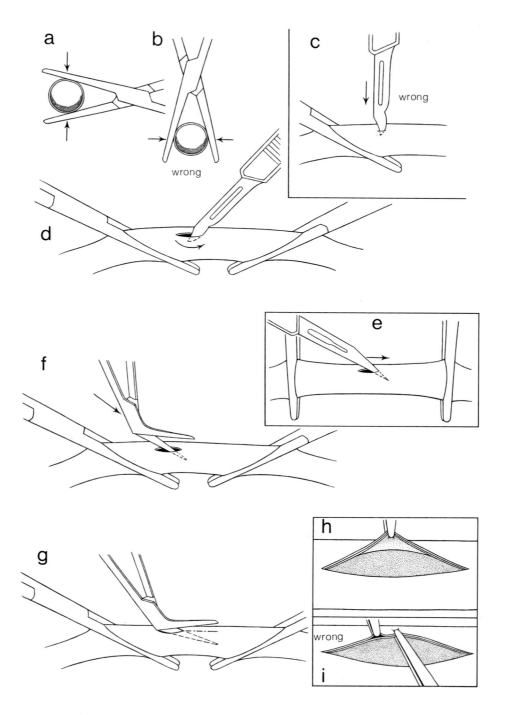

Figure 4-8. ARTERIOTOMY

forceps held by surgeon and assistant. Inserting closed forceps (blades approximated) through the arteriotomy site can separate edges. When edges must be grasped it is preferable to grasp all layers rather than to separate planes by handling only adventitia. Tension in blades of forceps influences the duration of careful holding of the vessel wall.

It is as important for the surgeon to practice a concept of precise needle handling as it is to have the wide array of sizes and configuration of needles and needle holders that are available. The effect of suturing is uniting tissues at a common point. Needle placement can make this junction precise, incorporating the desiderata of smooth surfaces and optimal strength. Penetrating all layers of the vessel wall equidistant from the arteriotomy site is essential. Deliberate direction of the needle point is achieved by aligning needle holder, hand, wrist, arm, and body so that the needle may pursue the intended course. The surgeon in training is fortunate if a thoughtful and articulate mentor describes, demonstrates, and insists upon adjustment of the surgeon to the task. There is no place for unplanned, inconsistent, imprecise, and arbitrary motions. There may be need for the discipline of correct practice any time any tissue is being sutured. Adaptation of excellence in concept and technique is applicable to vessels of most sizes in most sites. Maintained patency of reconstructions often depends upon caring enough to employ the very best surgeon and techniques.

Traction sutures to spread arteriotomy orifices are placed 3 to 5 mm from the cut edge of the artery, to preclude separation of plaque and wall and to avoid multiple needle holes at the site of the subsequent suture line. Traction sutures are placed two-thirds of the distance from the end at which suturing is started (Fig. 4-10).

Sutures are placed so that the needle point passes from the recipient vessel lumen to the outside, minimizing any tendency to separate plaque and wall. Sutures at each end of anastomoses between artery and graft are placed parallel to the direction of the arteriotomy incision, insuring that graft material will cover

---

Figure 4-8. Vertical or oblique application of arterial occluding clamps to vessels is the surgeon's tendency, since vessels lie at the depths of incisions. This may be wrong. At many sites of operation upon arteries there is varying thickness and brittleness of atheromata. The dorsal wall of abdominal aorta, iliac artery, and common femoral artery frequently harbor thick plaques. Least disturbance is caused by applying clamps in a manner that approximates the softer, yielding anterior wall against the nonpliable plaque wall (a).

Arterial incisions should enter lumina without separating the several layers of arterial wall. The incision is best started near one clamp (d), with consideration for ease of use of both scalpel and scissors. Deft entry of lumen (d, e) and single scissors-cut of precise length (g) may be better than plunging motion (c), which may injure the opposite wall. An incision thoughtlessly placed may require extension by multiple maneuvers.

Avoiding manipulation of wall is ideal. However, visibility adequate for operative maneuvers frequently requires handling of the vessel wall. The end-result is likely to be better when full-thickness of wall is handled (h) than when theoretically-good but practically-unsound technique of grasping adventitia (i, left) results in separation of layers. Then the end-result is likely to be ragged, thrombogenic intima and intramural separation conducive to anatomic deformity and nonlaminar flow.

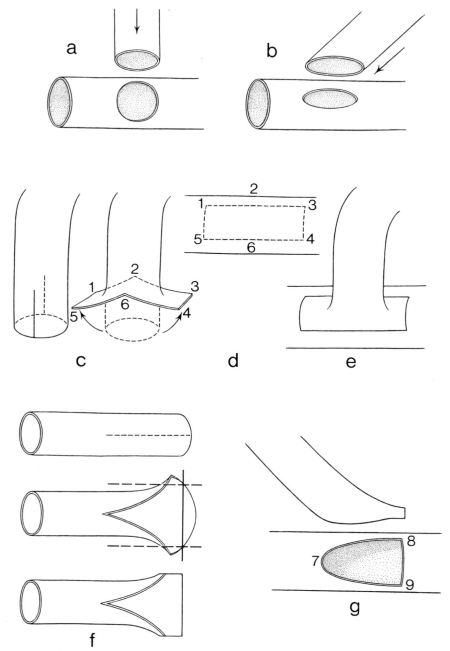

Figure 4-9. ARTERIOTOMY–BYPASS GRAFT VARIATIONS. Excision of a portion of wall of vessel assures ultimate diastolic dimensions of the orifice. Circular and elliptical junctions are common (a, b). Rectangular or eccentric "buttons" require specific preparation of ends of graft (c, f). A greater angle of incidence of graft may have to be assured with certain geometric configurations of anastomoses (e).

Suturing techniques must preclude purse-string effects. Two sutures (c: 1, 2, 3, 4 and c: 1, 5, 6, 4) may suffice, or the surgeon may prefer separate sutures to assure optimal diameter at transverse components of arteriotomy sites (d: 1, 5; d: 3, 4; and g: 8, 9).

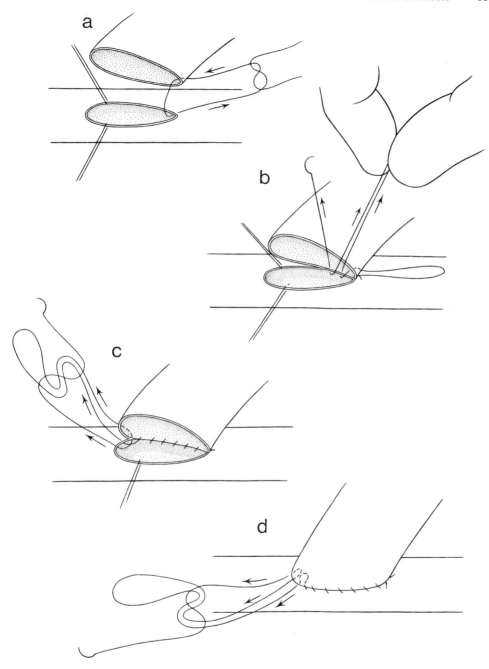

Figure 4-10.   BYPASS GRAFT. In contrast to simple closure, end-sutures must be placed beyond arteriotomy, for the inside of the graft is to abut the host intima (b, c) circumferentially. Suture direction is outside-in on the graft, inside-out on the host. Stay sutures are placed two-thirds to three-fourths of the distance from the site of initiating the anastomosis. Ideally, graft is made to overlie host wall as a peaked roof overhangs a wall. A second suture is used for the second 180° of anastomosis, and is *not* tied at either end to the previous suture. This precludes constriction.

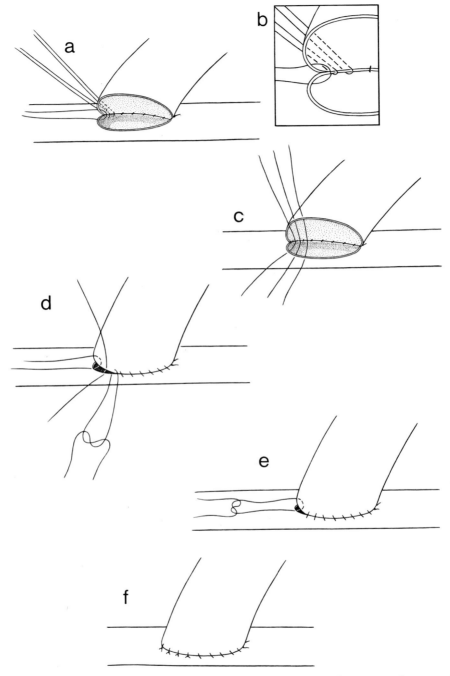

Figure 4-11. BYPASS GRAFT, SMALL ARTERY. Precise placement of a running suture gives way to placement of multiple interrupted sutures at distal end of graft-host vessel junction. These are not tied until the running suture on the second (near) side of arteriotomy has been placed and tied.

the end of the arteriotomy. Individual sutures on each side of the line of arteriotomy are used, for they retain the full circumference of recipient vessel at each end of the arteriotomy (Fig. 4-11). Mattress sutures are not used at the ends of arteriotomy sites; tying them may cause a constricting effect, and this must be avoided. The narrowest point of host vessel, not the widest segment of patch site, determines lumen size, blood flow capacity, and affects long-term patency.

Whether cloth or vein is employed as graft material, one cannot hope to appose precisely the cut edge of artery to the cut edge of graft. Consistent smooth transition can be effected by placing the inner wall of graft over the outer edge of artery wall, as a roof is applied over walls of a building. The edge of a graft nestles in the space between arteriotomy edge and extraluminal aspects of suture line.

CONCEPT AND TECHNIQUE AFFECTING RESULTS OF VESSEL ANASTOMOSES

When artery and graft are joined with continuous running suture, the suture rolls the graft lining inward, everts the wall of the artery, and compresses intima of graft to host at suture sites. Greater distances between sutures demand less tension to preclude shortening of the arteriotomy orifice or buckling (corrugating) effect upon host or graft vessel.

If the arteriotomy site is too long, simple closure may be effected, or an extra segment of cloth or vein may be tailored and incorporated into the graft-vessel junction.

If the bevel of the graft is disproportionately long, it may be trimmed, in preference to including larger amounts of graft between sutures. To preclude rolling excess graft wall or leaving excess potential space between host vessel and graft near the end of a line of anastomosis, the suture may be passed from outer wall of artery into lumen side (lining) of graft prior to tying. At the termination of a suture line, equal tension is placed on both limbs of the loop of suture material, assuring appropriate tension on the suture line and the knot. It is inadvisable to tie together the terminal ends of anastomosing sutures for the same reasons the initiating sutures were not joined—constriction is to be avoided; uniform caliber is sought to preclude turbulence and to permit optimal flow of blood.

Patch grafts are used with considerations concerning patterns of blood flow. Abrupt transitions in caliber alter laminar flow, promote turbulence, and encourage thrombosis. Whether cloth or vein is used, attention is directed to maintaining or gradually altering the caliber between vessels of disproportionate sizes at each end of the arteriotomy site. The purpose of a patch should be maintenance of optimum caliber to conform with known principles of hydraulics. Inspection and measurement of greatest diameters at midpoints of anastomoses of grafts (or angiograms of these areas) frequently disclose excesses compared to diameters of proximal and distal channels. Compensation is possible while anastomoses are in progress by placing sutures farther from the edges of arteriotomy and graft as the midpoint of this incision is approached.

ALLOGRAFTS

The appeal of artificial conduits includes the use of tissues from other people and even animals. When personal and recorded experience cite technical difficulties of tailoring and suturing woven or knitted materials to small sclerotic vessels in sites of limited accessibility, the use of supple animal tissue may be compelling. One must not forget that salvage procedures in high-risk patients are the issue. Homograft arterial substitutes had poor long-range results, but may have contributed appropriately in patients with end-stage systemic and local decompensation. The lesser content of muscle tissue of veins may minimize complications from the site that weakened most in arterial allografts. The lesser quantity of elastic tissue than in the aorta, which fared relatively well at five and ten years, may obviate the use of this base of comparison. Recorded experience at an average of one year, and up to two and one-half years, supports the use of allograft veins, especially when the alternative seems to be early failure for technical reasons.

Allografts appear indicated as arterial bypass grafts when rapid operating time with minimal trauma is desired, or when autogenous veins have been excised or are inflamed, fibrosed, or of inadequate caliber. Given the instance of absent or unsuitable saphenous veins, cephalic veins are not an automatic substitute without significant cosmetic disadvantage or technical travail. Limited distensibility of skin of forearm and of arm obligates the use of many small incisions or of unacceptable long incisions to remove the cephalic vein without local bleeding or occult traumatic disruption of vein wall integrity.

REOPERATION OF ARTERIES AT SITES OF PREVIOUS RECONSTRUCTION

The striking nature of change in the walls of arteries days, months, and years after operations upon them has not been emphasized (Fig. 4-12). For a few days after operation there is minimal difficulty in reconstructing an artery within a millimeter of the previous suture line. Transverse suture lines have appeared stronger than longitudinal. Later at reoperation, the surgeon may have technical difficulty because the media separates readily from the adventitia. This may be due to dense adherence between scar tissue that does not unite with the media despite becoming virtually integral with the adventitia. Sharp dissection onto the arterial wall within one centimeter of the suture line is safe if tension is not exerted at the suture line. Operation upon sites of weakness of reconstructed arterial walls is safest when approached deliberately through the lumen of the artery or graft. Of course, this requires preliminary isolation and control of vessels at a distance from suture lines. Limitations of exposure are imposed when a trifurcation is near the operative site. As an example, isolation of the profunda femoris artery is facilitated by appropriate exposure of proximal common femoral artery, superficial femoral artery, and bypass graft, permitting anterior traction which is not disruptive to the suture line. Then, dissection of the profunda at least a centimeter from its origin is preferable to risking inadvertent injury at the bifurcation. Alternatively, with control (occlusion) of the other arteries, inci-

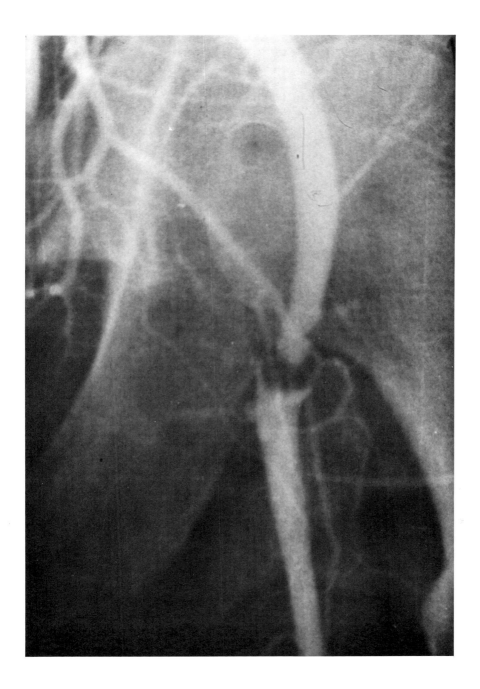

Figure 4-12. SHORT-SEGMENT OCCLUSION. Occlusion at femoral artery bifurcation at site of transverse arteriotomy for cannulation for cardiopulmonary bypass 7 months earlier. Filling of profunda by collateral circulation.

sion of the common femoral artery followed at once by insertion of a red rubber catheter of appropriate size can facilitate safe isolation of the profunda.

PROCEDURES IN ACUTE ISCHEMIA (EMBOLISM, THROMBOSIS)

Sudden reduction of blood flow to an extremity can induce symptoms and alter function. Peripheral nerves have a high metabolic requirement no longer satisfied after sudden arterial occlusion occurs. Inadequate delivery of oxygen and restrictive transport of metabolites cause parasthesias, altered sensitivity, subjective and objective changes in temperature, and reduced motor power. Examination discloses absence of pulses, altered hues and temperature, and diminished sensivity and motion. It is obvious that the abnormality may become catastrophic unless improvement is effected promptly. The patient must be admitted to the hospital at once for diagnosis and treatment. Meanwhile, extension of the process must be prevented by immediate administration of 75 mg of heparin intravenously, and collateral circulation must be promoted, comfort afforded, and differential diagnosis considered. The physician's suspicions must encompass more than certain well-known phenomena such as emboli in persons with rheumatic fever (whether or not atrial fibrillation is present) or following recent myocardial infarction (known or suspected).

Persons with atherosclerosis and diminished pulses at any site may have lesions which propagate thrombus proximally or distally. Diminished plasma volume (as a result of burns, vomiting, or increased red cell mass) predisposes to such thrombus formation. Young diabetics are prone to silent myocardial infarctions; prosthetic heart valves are the source of emboli in up to 30 percent of patients; arterioarterial emboli can occur in people with atherosclerosis.

Arterioarterial embolization has been given less attention than it deserves. Ulcerating atheromatous lesions of the aorta which predispose to thrombus formation are common; those in major arteries may be identified angiographically. A fragment of atheromatous plaque may become dislodged from a proximal nonoccluding or partially occluding lesion and be carried forward by arterial flow into a peripheral branch. Spontaneous forward propulsion of the embolus may occur if dissolution or fragmentation ensues. Collateral circulation can restore adequate though subnormal blood flow (Fig. 4-13). The diagnosis may be suspected in individuals with relative arterial insufficiency and proximal arterial lesions (e.g., moderate, unilateral intermittent claudication; differences in pulsations between the two sides; abnormal postural changes; prolonged venous filling time). It is dilatory to depend upon spontaneous restoration of adequate blood flow even though warmth, normal color, and line of demarcation extend distally. It is unacceptable to postulate that the combination of spontaneous improvement and conservative management is an effective substitute for intraluminal restoration of patency.

ANGIOGRAPHY BEFORE OPERATION. Angiography is important to identify unimpaired circulatory pathways distally which must have arterial blood flow restored whether occlusion is thrombotic or embolic in origin. Single exposure angiography is better than none, but it may fail to demonstrate information afforded by serial

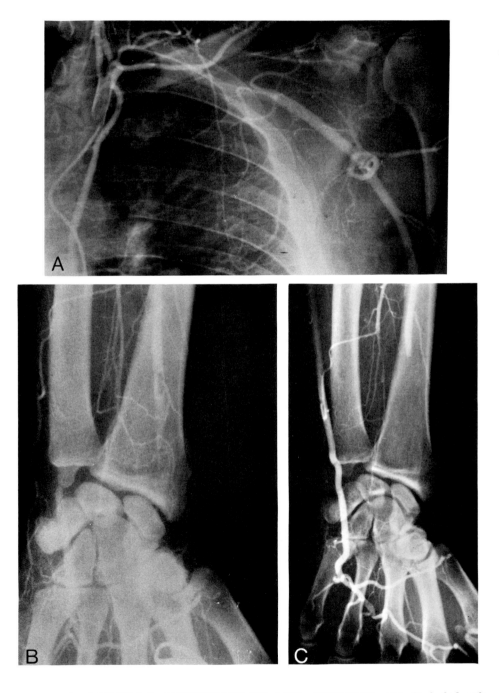

Figure 4-13. MULTIPLE OCCLUSIONS IN ARM ARTERIES. (A) Occluded subclavian artery, left, parts two and three, post-traumatic, with (B) thromboembolic oclusions of ulnar and distal radial arteries. (C) Final postoperative result (1965), prior to availability of Fogarty catheters.

angiography which is essential to evaluation and therapy. Angiography documents the clinical suspicion which operation may relieve.

Surgical restoration of mainline blood flow is preferred to waiting, in vain, for collateral circulation to effect disappearance of symptoms and signs and to restore circulation adequate for survival.

THE PRINCIPLE OF EMBOLECTOMY.   The goal of embolectomy is complete restoration of blood flow early enough to preserve tissue function. Circulation must be restored promptly through major and collateral vessels permitting blood to pass into arterioles, through capillaries, and into the venous system, to retain integrity of vascular walls and viability and function of muscles and nerves. Major vessels may be manipulated directly, while intramuscular and distal location of small arteries precludes direct operative intervention. Indirect removal of emboli is possible (see below) and may be preferred as the technique of clearing obstructions from small arteries.

ADVANTAGES OF INTRALUMINAL INSTRUMENTATION.   Three signs patently attest the need for mechanical dislodgement of adherent material from the walls of arteries: failure to restore blood flow, angiographic evidence of intraluminal irregularity, or early rethrombosis. When retrograde flush or balloon catheters (see below) have failed to restore patency, ureteral catheters of successively larger dimensions may be passed retrograde through an artery. The ingenious coiled wire instrument of Shaw or a catheter over which suture material has been wound have been found effective in removing adherent thrombus. A disadvantage is that this technique can remove portions of atheromata, a consequence of the abrasive effect of this coarse, channel-restoring instrumentation. Major deterrents to prolonged patency subsequently are incomplete removal of thrombus, traumatic denudation of vessel lining, and small caliber at site of arteriotomy repair. Low molecular weight dextran, heparin, and specific substances which diminish platelet adherence to vessel wall promote maintained patency in suboptimal conditions of arteries.

PRECISE USE AND LIMITATIONS OF BALLOON CATHETERS FOR EMBOLECTOMY.   The availability of Fogarty catheters has rekindled a laudable interest in embolectomy. Use of this catheter is not necessary if a single site of embolus permits operative exposure and embolectomy. Distal passage and withdrawal of the catheter may facilitate complete dislodgement of recent adherent thrombus from intima, and permit more complete removal of distal thrombus than is to be expected with aspiration. Thrombus material may be removed from proximal arteries (e.g., iliacs) and from prosthetic vessel grafts.

We employ Fogarty catheters when arteriotomy over the site of embolus is not feasible, when there are technical limitations to retrograde flush, when spasm must be overcome in an artery recently traumatized and thrombosed, and when red thrombus must be extruded from prosthetic grafts. Fogarty catheters are not used in lieu of a preferable procedure, nor as a mechanical probing substitute for knowledge better gained by angiography. Specifically, they should not be passed in all instances merely because it is easy to do.

ABUSES OF CONCEPTS OF EMBOLECTOMY AND THROMBECTOMY.   Passing a balloon catheter into distal vessels after successful local embolectomy is a maneuver without justification, for it may inflict intraluminal trauma with deleterious consequences. Embolus which is loosely lodged at a bifurcation may be impacted or fragmented as the catheter is passed distally. Withdrawal of a catheter may sheer one limb of a bifid embolus, failing to restore luminal continuity to all vessels. Residual embolic fragments not only obstruct other arteries but may be a focus upon which thrombus will reform in the vessel recently opened. The catheter cannot be expected to enter the anterior tibial artery when passed through a femoral or even proximal popliteal site. Passage into specific arteries (e.g., peroneal, anterior or posterior tibial) is accomplished with certainty by surgical exposure of these vessels distal to the knee (see Fig. 4-15).

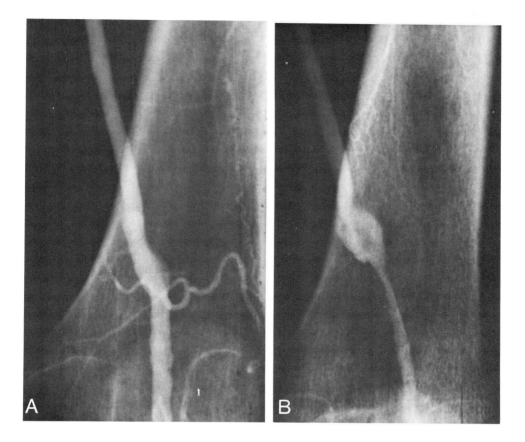

Figure 4-14. POSTOPERATIVE ANGIOGRAPHIC EVALUATION. (A) Uniform caliber at anastomosis site. (B) False aneurysm causing extraluminal compression of vein graft and clamp defect at distal end of anastomosis. Angiograms at operation can disclose clamp trauma. Angiograms several days after opertion can disclose remediable faults early enough to correct them with least monetary or functional deficit.

ANGIOGRAPHY AT OPERATION. Angiography in operating rooms has shown its usefulness just as routine visualization after arterial reconstruction and embolectomy has demonstrated its value. It is a worthwhile adjunct to procedures already employed—careful surgical technique, release of clamps immediately before completing suture lines, palpation of pulse distally, and recording of blood flow. Operative angiograms have demonstrated unanticipated but significant correctable abnormalities. Unsuspected emboli have been removed from distal small vessels which are vital to organ function. Narrowed lumina caused by incompletely removed atheromata, thrombus, imprecise technique of reconstruction, or previously unrecognized intramural dissections have been enlarged (Figs. 4-14 and 4-15). Remediable kinks, dilatations, and turbulent flow at locations of patch grafts have been recognized (Fig. 4-16). The need for careful surgical technique has been demonstrated by angiographic evidence of damage of intima of artery from clamps and tapes placed proximal and/or distal to the site of arteriotomy. Defects secondary to extraluminal compression or discrepancies of length and caliber of graft

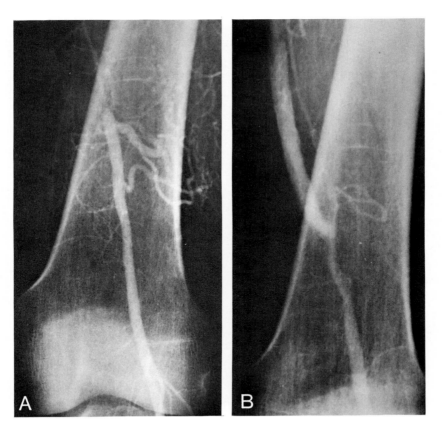

Figure 4-15. ROUTINE POSTOPERATIVE ANGIOGRAPHY. (A) Angiogram shows major collateral vessels filling popliteal artery distal to segmental occlusion of superficial femoral artery. (B) Postoperative angiogram disclosed significant stenosis of popliteal artery distal and proximal to site of implantation of graft, and nonfilling of larger, superior collateral artery.

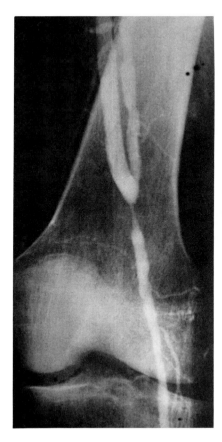

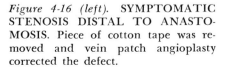

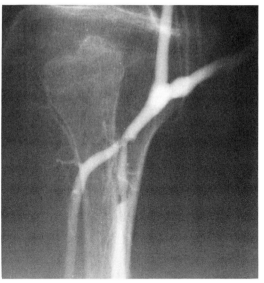

Figure 4-17 (right). CLAMP TRAUMA. This routine postoperative angiogram shows all too common lesion of clamp trauma distal to site of anastomosis. The density of contrast medium in host (popliteal) artery proximal to anastomosis indicates lesser resistance preferential flow, implying functional obstruction by iatrogenic defect. Intramural clot as well as thrombogenic surface will hasten thrombosis.

Use of intraluminal stents during operation will preclude this type of defect. Operative angiography permits detection and correction at once. The routine of postoperative angiography compels correction or resignation to suboptimal result, and explains early thrombosis postoperatively.

Figure 4-16 (left). SYMPTOMATIC STENOSIS DISTAL TO ANASTO-MOSIS. Piece of cotton tape was removed and vein patch angioplasty corrected the defect.

material have been evident. Abnormal communications or obstructions which threaten function in in-situ vein grafts used for arterial bypass may not be apparent to observation without angiography. Extent of obliteration of arteriovenous fistulas has been documented.

Postoperative angiography may supplant ignorance, prejudices, and differences of opinion among surgeons, by explaining, avoiding, and correcting causes of failure of maintained patency of reconstructed arteries (Figs. 4-17 and 4-18). Similar abnormalities may be induced by varieties of techniques, and angiography may demonstrate this conclusively. Reconstructed vessels with architecture demonstrated conducive to prolonged patency have yielded predictably favorable clinical courses. Newer surgical concepts need not suffer unfair criticism when angiography is a principal arbiter.

Appropriate precautions for angiography in any region of the body are always in order (e.g., hydration, placement of needle, selection and quantity of contrast substance). Angiography does not complicate nor unduly prolong operations if preparation has been made for it.

Unpreparedness is a state of mind, raising the question of the propriety of performing time-consuming major vascular operations without complete mobilization of those same resources mandatory for preoperative diagnosis, and for assessing results or complications out of the operating suite. The many instances of routine use and usefulness of operative angiography refute any protestations of impracticality, cost or needlessness.

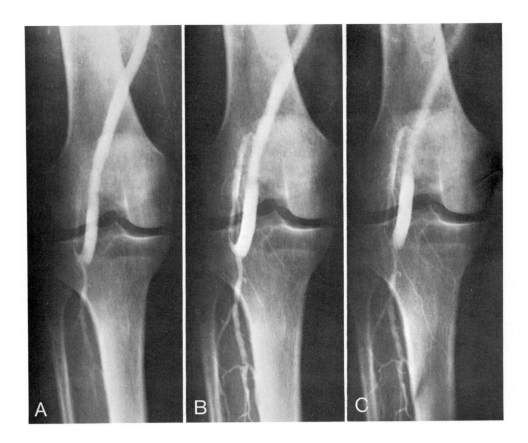

Figure 4-18.   ADVANTAGES OF SERIAL ANGIOGRAPHY. A principal thesis of this book is that *each* detail is *the* most important one. Figure A demonstrates and C corroborates abnormalities of structure and function that will limit the duration of patency and effectiveness of flow consequent to technical imperfection of reconstructive (bypass) operation. Figure A discloses marked density of contrast medium in graft, secondary to relative obstruction to flow through small residual lumen at site of anastomosis. These facts are obscured in B, but the delay in flow from graft to host vessel is emphasized again in C.

REGIONAL SURGICAL MANAGEMENT

CAROTID-VERTEBRAL ARTERIES

Extracranial arteries.   Extensive experience correlating clinical neurology with pathologic anatomy visualized by three-dimensional angiography has emphasized three points: atherosclerotic involvement of extracranial and intracranial distributions of carotid and vertebral arteries is diffuse; neurologic history and findings correspond with demonstrated arterial pathology in 80 percent of instances; and neurologic abnormalities exist without demonstrable vascular lesions in expected locations in 20 percent of patients. Arterial reconstruction of extracranial stenoses of carotid or vertebral arteries relieves symptoms in half the symptomatic patients and prevents progression in one-third, but it is associated with complications, persistence of symptoms, or death in up to 15 percent of patients. Heart and brain have shared equally in consequences and causes of morbidity and mortality.

Symptoms of ischemia of the brain demand angiography to detect remediable obstructive causes in carotid and vertebral arteries. Cerebral angiography performed with general anesthesia has had no higher incidence of complications than when performed with local anesthesia. When neurosurgeons perform angiography routinely after clipping an intracranial aneurysm, effects of contrast media have not created a higher incidence of complications. Stenoses greater than 50 percent of the diameter of the extraosseous portion of the vertebral artery or of the extracranial portion of carotid arteries are considered indications for operation. Total occlusion of the internal carotid artery may be reopened permanently in 25 to 40 percent of instances. Ulcerating lesions of atheromata, identifiable on angiograms as irregularities or craters, require operation even though they constrict lumina less than 50 percent. They are hazardous as thrombogenic surfaces, and craters imply discharge of semisolid matter from plaque into the bloodstream (arterioarterial embolism). Hemorrhage into and beneath plaques may occur at ulcerated sites, further narrowing the arterial lumen (Fig. 4-19).

Contraindications to operation of the carotid artery are total occlusion with evidence of progressive infarction and bloody cerebrospinal fluid. A current working hypothesis obviates operation until after the fourteenth day following strokes. Vertebral artery reconstruction is hazardous technically when advanced atherosclerotic involvement of the subclavian artery coexists. Application of clamps to the subclavian artery can fracture plaques, create dissections of arterial wall, and result in thrombosis of the subclavian-vertebral system. Multiple sites of stenoses limit the likelihood of markedly increasing total flow to brain unless all sites are reconstructed. Contralateral occlusion of the carotid artery limits blood flow to the brain during operative arterial occlusion. Operations requiring transient occlusions of the only functioning carotid artery may be done safely with appropriate adjuncts to increase cerebral blood flow and monitoring methods which assure adequacy of circulation to the brain. Cervical block anesthesia, elevated P_{CO_2}, EEG monitoring of response to arterial occlusion, and intra-arterial shunt all may be necessary. Suspected embolization to the brain rarely has been

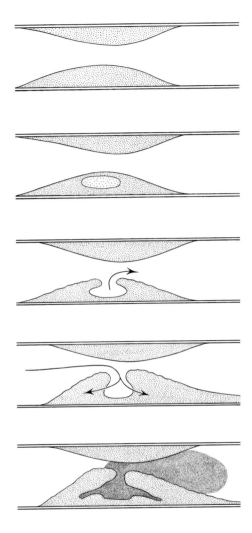

Figure 4-19. PATHOPHYSIOLOGY OF ULCERATED PLAQUE. Commonly plaques which do not narrow lumen significantly cause central nervous system symptoms from extruded atheromatous material. The crater in the atheroma is excessively thrombogenic. Systolic and diastolic thrusts can initiate intramural expansion of atheroma, significantly narrowing lumen, slowing blood flow, resulting in thrombosis. (See also Fig. 3-3).

followed by aggressive diagnostic radiologic or surgical procedures. Responses to carbon dioxide and to time have brought discernible rapid improvement so frequently that physicians have been content to do nothing more, despite residual deficits. Anticoagulation has been started promptly to preclude reformation of thrombus at the source of embolus. Angiographic evidence of ulcerating atheromatous plaques in carotid arteries has been sought when fundoscopic examination disclosed fibrin or cholesterol, for ulcerating plaque has been interpreted as an indication for early operation.

Carotid endarterectomy.   Carotid endarterectomy requires use of the usual principles of arterial surgery—gentle circumferential mobilization of the main artery and its branches, systemic administration of heparin, and application of noncrushing clamps several millimeters distal to the proposed limits of the arteriotomy (Figs. 4-20 to 4-24). The internal carotid artery is clamped first, to preclude passage of intra-arterial debris, as other clamps are applied to vessels with their atheromata which not uncommonly extend cephalad on the dorsal wall of the internal carotid artery. Anterior rotation of clamps prior to arteriotomy permits incision in the lateral wall of the artery, with that aspect directly in view. Lateral incision affords an excellent view and perspective of the relation of the atheroma to the orifice of the external carotid artery. The incision is carried five millimeters proximal and distal to the principal plaque. The plane between the mature atheroma and the media commonly presents itself and is readily developed with a freer elevator. Circumferential isolation and division of the plaque is achieved distal and proximal to the orifice of the external carotid artery. A 360 degree view of the origin of the latter permits sharp termination of dissection of the plaque of the external carotid artery. The bulk of the atheroma is removed. Traction upon the wall of the common carotid artery permits incision of the intima with fine-pointed sharp scissors, delineating the proximal extent of endarterectomy of residual plaque. A similar incision terminates dissection into the internal carotid artery. If the plaque of the external carotid artery must be removed, a separate incision in that artery permits termination of endarterectomy with complete visibility and precise technique. Arteriotomy sites are closed with continuous fine suture material, 5-0 silk, polyethylene, or tycron. Sutures are not placed beyond the ends of arteriotomy sites; they include 0.5 to 1 mm of wall, and are 1 to 1.5 mm apart. Prior to placing or tightening sutures in the final 3 mm of arterial closure, back-bleeding from internal and external carotid arteries is permitted, and a clamp is placed proximal to the bifurcation, allowing internal and external artery flow. Prior to releasing the clamp on the common carotid artery, the clamp proximal to the bifurcation is moved to the origin of the internal carotid artery. After blood is flowing from common to external, the internal carotid artery is unclamped.

If an internal shunt is used (Figs. 4-25 to 4-27), a 4-inch length of tubing 4 mm in diameter is employed (plastic tubing or infusion set). A 2-0 ligature is tied an inch from one end, and a small hemostat grasps this ligature. Narrow umbilical tapes are passed around the internal and common carotid arteries, and occluding clamps are placed proximal and distal to the tapes. Incision is made in the com-

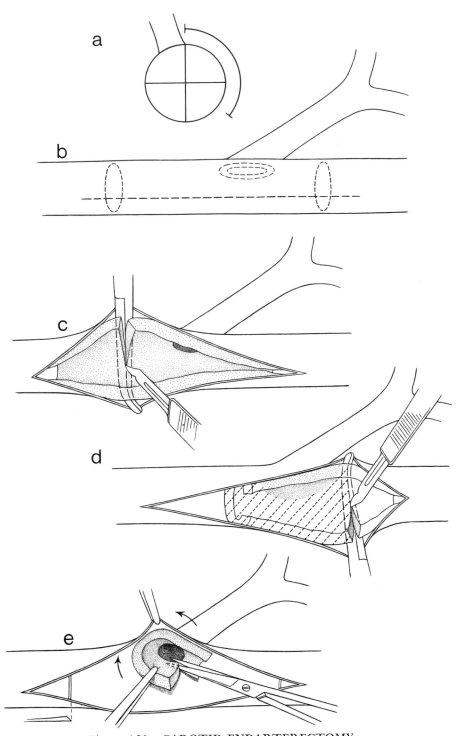

Figure 4-20.   CAROTID ENDARTERECTOMY

Figures 4-20 and 4-21. CAROTID ENDARTERECTOMY. Incision in posterolateral wall of common and internal carotid arteries is placed 120° from origin of external carotid artery, and extends beyond proximal and distal portions of plaque. A freer elevator may be needed to initiate the plane of dissection (Fig. 4-20) which is continued with a right angle clamp. The bulk of the plaque is readily excised (cross-hatched area), improving visibility for careful incision of plaque of tributary artery. It is important to not separate tributary plaque from attachment to its wall, and to terminate endarterectomy in carotid arteries precisely in full view (Fig. 4-21).

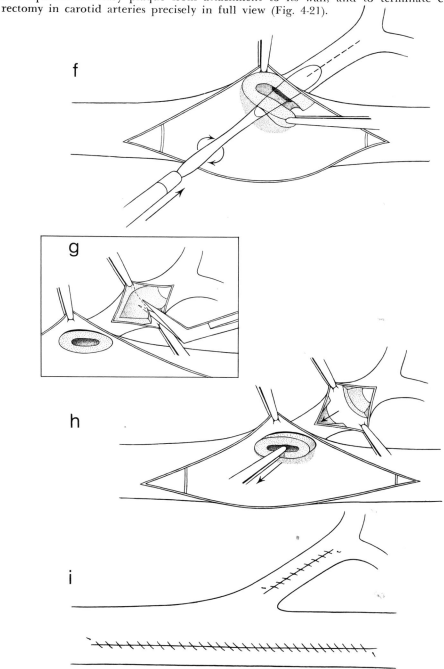

mon and internal arteries. The 3-inch segment of tubing is passed into the internal carotid artery as an assistant releases the occluding clamp and tightens the tape. When back-bleeding fills the shunt, it is clamped. The proximal 1-inch segment is inserted into the common carotid artery, the shunt clamps removed, and the proximal tape tightened. The proximal clamp is removed. The marking ligature around the shunt is clamped to the proximal tape to stabilize the position of the shunt tube.

A number of *incorrect maneuvers are to be avoided.* Manipulation against the artery prior to occlusion may loosen embolic material (e.g., platelets, atheromata, debris). Traction exerted on the edges of the incised atheroma may disengage the atheromatous plaque as it enters the external carotid artery, or as it continues in attenuated lamina onto the posterior wall of the internal carotid artery. It is important to tailor residual intima or thin layers of atheromatous lining, so thrombogenic surfaces do not exist. Subintimal dissection of the plaque may occur during systole and diastole in proximal and distal portions of the artery unless the intima and media are in apposition. Tacking sutures, no matter how they are placed, are less effective in preventing thrombosis than is optimal endarterectomy technique.

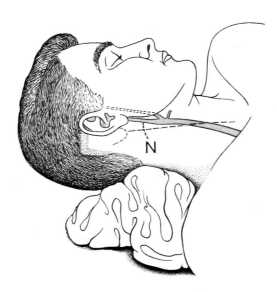

Figure 4-22. CONCEPTS AND LANDMARKS TO EXPOSE BIFURCATION OF CAROTID ARTERY. Area shaved is shown. Drapes exclude ear from operative field. Palpate the mastoid process. Incision proceeds along anterior border of sternocleidomastoid muscle, stopping 4 cm from clavicle. Great auricular nerve (N) must not be cut. (Bifurcation of carotid artery is caudad of line projecting posteriorly from inferior ramus of mandible.)

In principle and practice, tissues are dissected from the arteries, to avoid manipulation of atheroma and possible thrombi at the bifurcation. The hypoglossal nerve is protected from injury by dissecting of internal carotid artery along its posterolateral aspects; this visualizes the nerve without touching it.

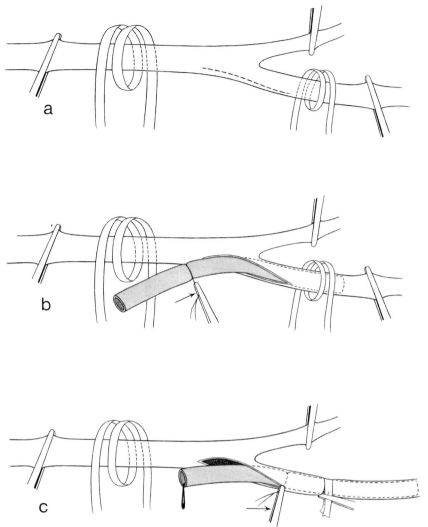

Figure 4-23. INTERNAL SHUNT FOR CAROTID ARTERY SURGERY. (a) Tapes are passed twice around common and internal carotid arteries (to hold shunt tubing), and external carotid is clamped, preparatory to lateral placement of clamps on internal, then common carotid arteries, distal and proximal to tapes. (Application of vascular clamps is not without hazard of fracturing intima-atheroma, and reapplication or multiple applications magnify the risk of fragmenting the lining or creating a thrombogenic surface or site of entry for intramural dissection.) Anteromedial rotation of clamps permits incision 120 degrees from bifurcation, which provides optimum exposure for endarterectomy, minimizes likelihood of unwanted intramural dislocation of residual plaque of external carotid artery, and provides wide cuff of artery to facilitate suture closure.

(b) Incision extends across atheromatous narrowing of artery. Shunt tube 4 inches long with ligature tied 1½ inches from protruding end is advanced into internal carotid artery. Tape is tightened around internal carotid artery and tube prior to releasing clamp on internal carotid artery. Tube is clamped near ligature as air is displaced by backbleeding.

(c) Internal shunt tube has been inserted to ligature, and is ready to be passed proximally into common carotid artery.

Figure 4-24. INTERNAL SHUNT FOR CAROTID ARTERY SURGERY. (d) Back-bleeding from internal carotid artery is allowed to displace air from shunt tube and segment of common carotid artery between tape and clamp, as proximal clamp is released and blood flow restored from common through internal carotid arteries. A hemostat remains applied to the ligature on the shunt tube as a visual reminder of its proper location, to prevent displacement during endarterectomy.

(e) After completion of endarterectomy (see Figs. 4-1, 4-2, 4-20, and 4-21), primary or patch closure, begun on internal carotid artery, proceeds onto common carotid artery.

(f) Assistants release clamp on external carotid artery and the tape around internal carotid artery as shunt is withdrawn, and common carotid artery is clamped proximal to bifurcation. This communication of flow between external and internal carotid arteries contributes to intracranial circulation and oxygenation as the residual arteriotomy is closed. The proximal clamp is released transiently, allowing air to escape through the arteriotomy site, and reapplied.

(g) The distal clamp on the common carotid artery is removed and applied obliquely on the internal carotid artery, directing blood flow into external carotid territory as the proximal clamp is removed permanently. This is intended to flush any intravascular debris away from the brain. Caution is cited concerning application of clamps across sutures (f, g). To prevent weakening or cutting of suture material, the clamps must be broad-toothed, soft-biting, and lightly applied.

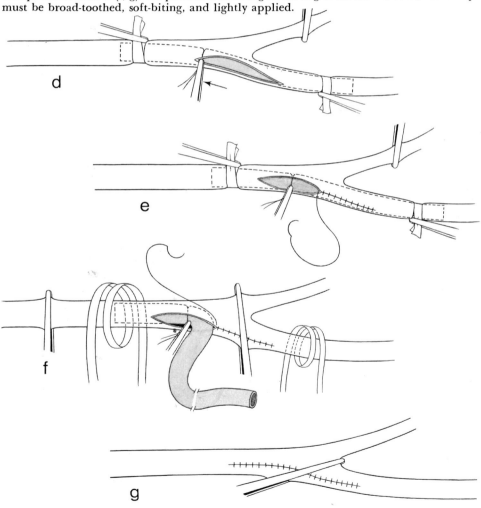

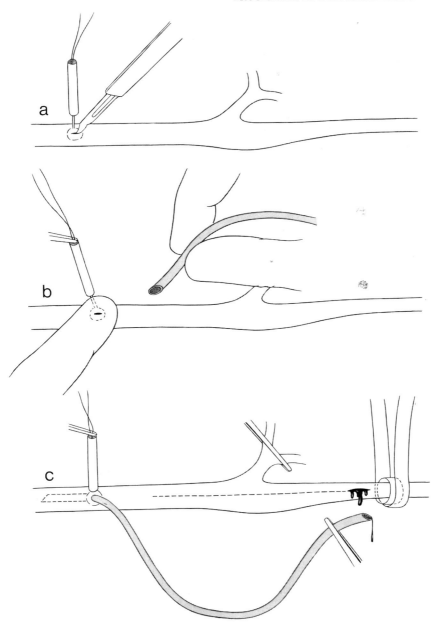

Figure 4-25. INTERNAL ARTERIAL SHUNT WITHOUT INTERRUPTION OF FLOW. Carotid arteries are depicted, and isolation of vessels, tape around internal carotid, and preparation for clamping external carotid artery distal to bifurcation proceed as in Figure 4-23. However, flow through common carotid artery will not be interrupted until shunt is functioning. Small "bites" of 4-0 suture material through adventitia and media are placed for first assistant's manipulation as stab wound arteriotomy (b) is controlled by digital pressure preparatory to insertion of proximal portion of shunt tube (c). With blood filling the tube, a stab wound is placed beyond atheroma to receive distal end of shunt and flow through it. (Ligatures around shunt tubing, as in Figure 4-24, may be placed as indicators and stabilizers of position of shunt.)

Figure 4-26. INTERNAL ARTERIAL SHUNT WITHOUT INTERRUPTION OF FLOW. Endarterectomy completed (as in Fig. 4-6), a second shunt tube is placed through arteriotomy of tributary (e). The principal arteriotomy is closed subtotally, to a point that permits arterial clamping proximal to the location of the second shunt tubing (f). A double-male adapter in place on the second tubing permits prompt union of withdrawn primary shunt tube. (This takes less time than tying previously placed interrupted sutures at proximal site of main arterial incision). When main arteriotomy has been closed, clamp is removed. (This seemingly complex maneuvering can preclude any interruption of flow, and minimizes time of transient decrease in intracranial arterial pressure or flow.) Purse-string suture on carotid artery is tied as shunt tube is withdrawn. Tributary artery (external carotid) is clamped transiently for suturing after removal of its shunt tube.

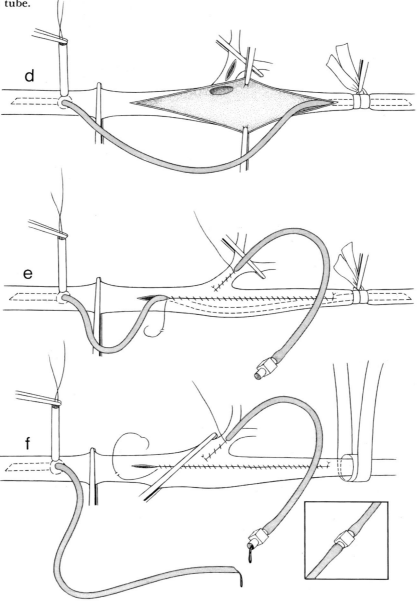

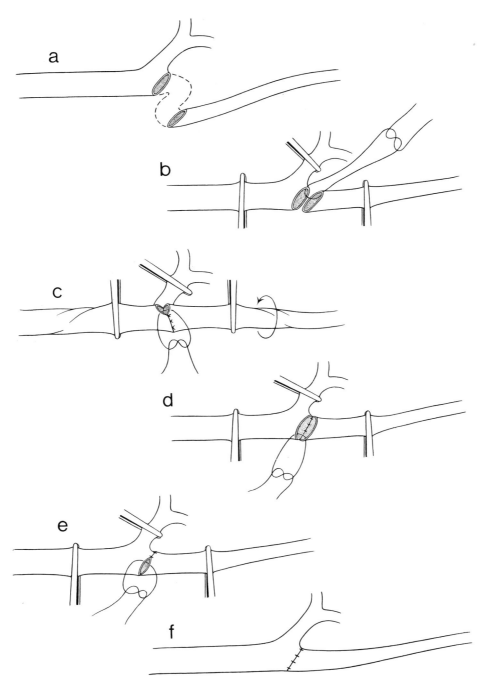

Figure 4-27. REMOVAL AND RECONSTRUCTION OF ELONGATED, KINKED ARTERY. Carotid arteries frequently are elongated. Removal of internal rigidity of the atheroma may accentuate the kink, making resection advisable. Disproportion in cross-sectional area may be minimized by bevels of different angles and by placement of interrupted sutures. Closure of the "back wall" is facilitated by 180° rotation of clamps.

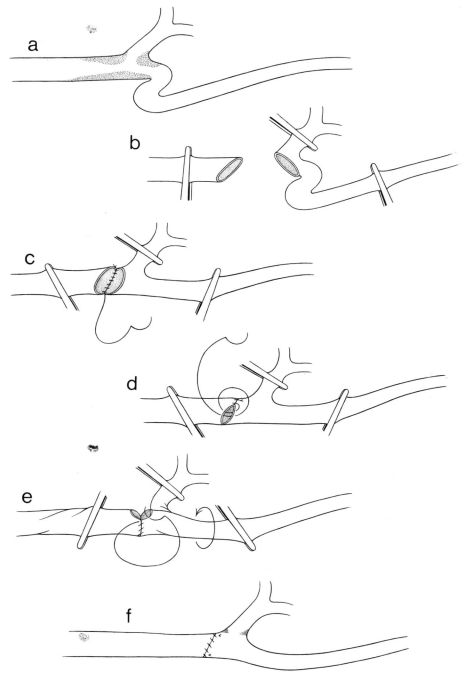

Figure 4-28. EXCISION OF SEGMENT OF PARENT ARTERY TO RELIEVE KINK IN TRIBUTARY. Bevelled removal of segment of common carotid artery prepares way for reconstruction without kink. Maneuvers of clamps and technique of suturing are similar to those in Figure 4-27, but the larger dimensions of arteries permit use of continuous suture technique. If preference or conditions warrant closure from outside of artery, rotation of clamps and artery facilitates this (e).

Elongation of the common and internal carotid arteries occurs. The external carotid artery may serve as a pivot point, kinking the proximal portion of the internal carotid artery. Excision and end-to-end anastomosis of the internal carotid artery seems an unacceptable routine because of the time it takes and technical complications which may be caused. Wedge excision of the common carotid artery and reconstruction of the large caliber artery is likely to be successful (Figs. 4-28). Plicating sutures may reduce the kink. A composite reconstruction, enlarging the lumen size at the kink site, may reduce the impediment to flow, though turbulence remains. Onlay patches of cloth or vein require separate sutures on each side that are not tied to each other across the end of arteriotomy sites.

Elongation of the proximal, extraosseous portion of the vertebral artery in atherosclerosis is common (Fig. 4-29). Such elongation facilitates improved techniques of relieving atherosclerotic stenoses and correcting kinks of this artery (Figs. 4-30 and 4-31). The excessive length of the vertebral artery permits ligation and division proximally. It is then joined to the subclavian artery or the thyrocervical axis at a site laterally in the wound that is technically more convenient for anastomosis. Improved exposure and use of vessels less affected by atherosclerosis favors precise surgical technique and assures prolonged patency of the reconstruction. Finally, there is greater safety and ease of surgical manipulation when the subclavian artery is not dissected proximal to the origin of the vertebral artery.

The subclavian and vertebral arteries are exposed via incision above and parallel to the clavicle, dividing the lateral head of the sternocleidomastoid muscle. The phrenic nerve is mobilized from the anterior scalene muscle, and the latter is freed from the subclavian artery and divided. A tape is passed around the subclavian artery medial to the thyrocervical axis preparatory to anastomosis to the vertebral artery. Areolar tissue obscuring the course of the vertebral artery to the transverse processes of lower cervical vertebrae is separated to locate and isolate the vertebral artery. Its site of ligation and division is made from an estimate of the length of distal vertebral artery necessary for anastomosis to the thyrocervical axis (end-to-end) or to the subclavian artery (end-to-side).

Heparin is given intravenously before the vertebral artery is ligated with 2-0 silk, clamped distally, and divided. The thyrocervical trunk is ligated proximal to its branches to permit circulation through the common stump, and it is clamped and divided near the subclavian artery. Interrupted sutures of 5-0 silk or polyethylene are placed circumferentially, then tied, uniting the vertebral artery to an uncompromised subclavian source. Closure is effected without drainage.

When the carotid artery is treated surgically at the same operation and prior to vertebral artery replantation, the oblique incision along the anterior border of the sternocleidomastoid muscle may be curved laterally just above the clavicle, providing exposure for operation upon the vertebral artery (Fig. 4-32).

Disarticulation or division of the clavicle has not been considered necessary in operative reconstruction of lesions of the origin of the vertebral artery. This improved exposure does not obviate certain disadvantages which may occur when operating upon the junction of vertebral and subclavian arteries. Horner's syndrome may be caused by trauma of vigorous, prolonged retraction upon cervical

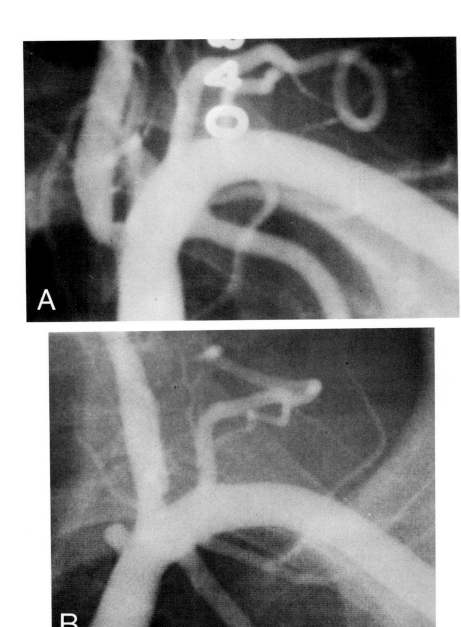

Figure 4-29.   VERTEBRAL ARTERY ABNORMALITIES CORRECTED BY OPERA-
TION. (A) LAO view of origin of vertebral artery from left subclavian artery. Elongation,
stenosis of origin, post-stenotic dilatation, and kinking, evident in A, have been corrected
by reimplantation laterally (B, AP view).

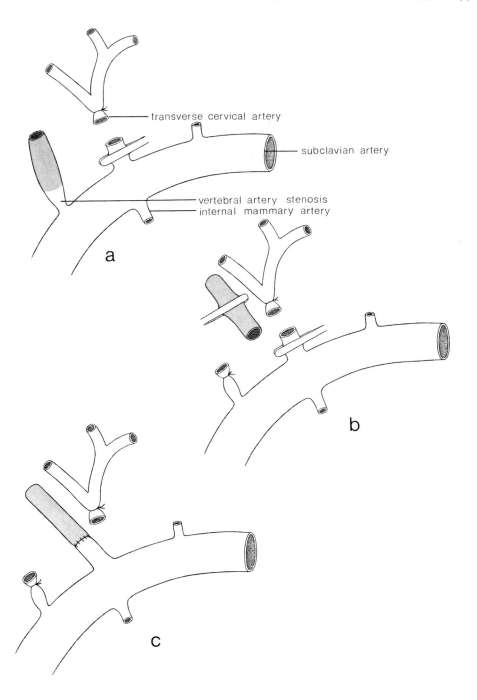

Figure 4-30. TRANSPOSITION OF VERTERBRAL ARTERY. (a) Thyrocervical axis has been clamped proximally, preparatory to anastomosis with vertebral artery. (b) Vertebral artery has been ligated, clamped, and divided, and is being moved laterally for anastomosis. (c) Completed anastomosis between vertebral artery and thyrocervical axis.

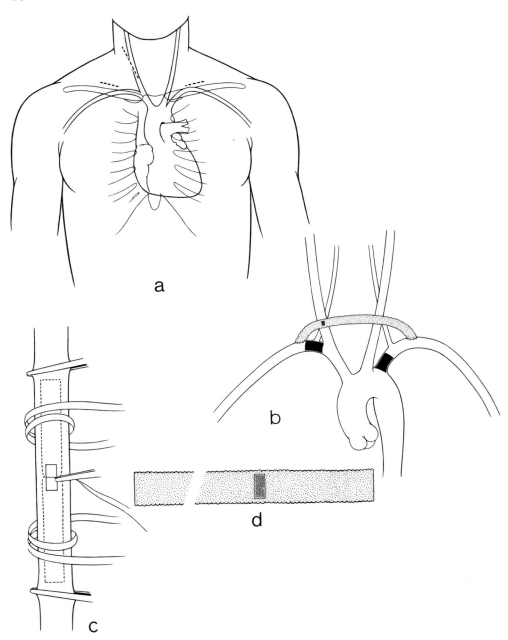

Figure 4-31. CAROTID-SUBCLAVIAN CROSSOVER BYPASS. (a) Standard incisions for exposure of common carotid artery and subclavian arteries are depicted. Tunnels beneath sternocleidomastoid muscles and across midline permit placement of graft (b). This drawing illustrates the sites of occlusions of subclavian arteries bilaterally in patient with claudication in arms. There was no history consistent with "carotid-subclavian steal syndrome." (c) Internal shunt is placed. This is similar to techniques illustrated in Figures 4-23 to 4-26. (d) A window created in anterior wall of common carotid artery determines the size of aperture created in cloth graft. The graft will be turned, apposing orifices.

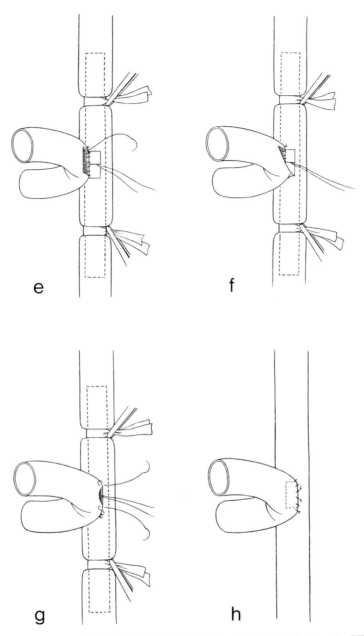

Figure 4-32. CAROTID-SUBCLAVIAN CROSSOVER BYPASS (cont.). The internal shunt is functioning (e, f). One suture unites a long and a transverse component of host-graft orifices. (g) A second suture approximates the second transverse component of aperture, and part of longitudinal cut. A third suture starts toward middle of remaining opening. (h) It becomes necessary to clamp carotid artery transiently to remove shunt. Then the two sutures close the defect and are tied to themselves (not to each other). Flow through carotid artery is restored and flow into graft is initiated. Pressure in graft distends it and aids correct estimate of its length, prior to suturing into place in each subclavian artery (Fig. 4-31, b).

sympathetic ganglia. Disruption of the subclavian artery or its branches is a possibility, although this has not been observed. Fracture of plaques resulting in intramural dissection and occlusion of the subclavian artery can occur. Difficulty dissecting a thumb-tack plaque from the subclavian artery or terminating its dissection smoothly inside the vertebral artery is to be avoided. Incision across the junction of the subclavian and vertebral arteries and prolonged operation of onlay patch graft are circumvented by implantation at a lateral site (see Fig. 4-29, p. 94). Elimination of causes of symptoms due to elongation, tortuosity, and kinks are inherent in this technique.

It should be apparent on preoperative angiograms if an embolus obstructs the vertebral artery orifice, and supraclavicular isolation of the extraosseous portion of the vertebral artery is indicated to obviate central embolization. Longitudinal incision in the subclavian artery 90 degrees away from the origin of the vertebral artery permits embolectomy. Spontaneous expulsion of the embolus is desirable, for it will remain intact and will remove adherent thrombus simultaneously. The supraclavicular approach to the subclavian artery is not well-tolerated with local anesthesia. Local complications of operation upon the vertebral artery via the subclavian artery may be expected to be minimal.

A longitudinal incision in the proximal portion of the vertebral artery, continued transversely onto the subclavian artery, may be reconstructed with a patch. Distal to its orifice, the vertebral artery may be divided to accomplish endarterectomy or to shorten the artery and reunited with six or more interrupted sutures. Plication has been advocated to remove kinks.

ARTERIES OF THE ARM

Subclavian artery. Embolus to the subclavian artery may obstruct its origin or may lodge at the trifurcation of vertebral-internal mammary branches, or farther distally. Central nervous symptoms may be evident when there are deficiencies of circulation through other arteries to the brain. Arm symptoms and signs are the least menacing that may occur. The arm may be highly symptomatic, but not often is viability threatened. Coldness and parasthesias are disturbing to patients; pain and weakness are not prominent. Examination above the medial aspect of the clavicle, adjacent to the lateral head of the sternomastoid, may disclose a pulse even if the obstruction is at the origins of the vertebral and internal mammary arteries, but not if the orifice of the subclavian artery has been obstructed. Occasionally there are advanced atherosclerotic processes in the subclavian artery where it is crossed by the anterior scalene muscle, and the embolus may be trapped at that level.

In the context of systemic disease responsible for both embolus to the subclavian artery and suboptimal physiologic status of patient, it may be preferable to complete diagnostic studies prior to thoracotomy to relieve obstruction at the origin of the subclavian artery. Cardiopulmonary disease and recent myocardial infarction may be relative contraindications to operation. Rheumatic heart disease may require assessment of severity of stenoses and regurgitation at multiple valve sites by cardiac catheterization to permit correction of intracardiac lesions at the same operation.

Embolic obstruction at the orifice of the left subclavian artery may demonstrate an "iceberg phenomenon" with a component in the aorta that requires aortotomy for removal. If angiography discloses contrast substance in the initial millimeters of the subclavian artery, the aorta need not be mobilized or clamped. The subclavian artery is gently mobilized, and if inspection and palpation do not suggest obstruction at origins of its branches, the branches need not be controlled. Transverse or longitudinal arteriotomy over the embolus is satisfactory, the proximal extent of the incision ending one centimeter from the aorta, permitting clamping of the subclavian artery after the embolus extrudes itself or is pulled out with a balloon catheter.

There are hazards of distal embolization if an embolus with an aortic component is manipulated; accordingly, neither traction nor balloon catheter is used. Rather, a partially excluding vascular clamp is placed on the aorta to contain the embolus within the site of incision.

Distal passage of a catheter perfunctorily into branches of the subclavian artery is not done. If distal pulses are not restored, the vertebral artery is occluded prior to attempts to aspirate or extract the embolus from the subclavian, axillary, and brachial arteries.

Brachial artery. Untreated emboli to axillary and brachial arteries have less serious prognoses since the greater collateral circulation around the axillary artery assures viability of arm and hand. The current ease and safety of angiography and embolectomy of the subclavian artery and all segments distal to it demand their use in treating occlusion of arteries to the arm. Thus, absence of pulse in an upper extremity is cause for angiogram and decision regarding site of operation. The proximal brachial artery is exposed with local anesthesia, and incision medial to the biceps muscle is extended along the inferior aspect of the pectoral fold of the axilla. Nerves are readily identified, mobilized minimally, and spared. The brachial artery is isolated proximal and distal to the origin of the circumflex humerus artery. Heparin administration is continued or is given intravenously, and longitudinal incision is made in the brachial artery. After assuring back-bleeding from the major artery and its tributary, a balloon catheter is passed proximally, *never as far as the vertebral artery,* and the catheter and inflated balloon are withdrawn. Often there is loosening of thrombus and embolus as withdrawal of the balloon catheter is started, and partial deflation of the balloon as withdrawal continues results in extrusion of obstructing material by arterial pressure. The proximal artery is clamped, arteriotomy site closed, and distal pulses evaluated. If brachial pulse at the elbow and radial pulse at the wrist are not palpable and if preoperative angiography had demonstrated patency, spasm is the presumed cause. It may be overcome promptly by transient reocclusion of the artery, and pulsatile injection into distal brachial artery of 50 cc of warm saline containing 10 cc of 1 percent procaine. Release of the arterial clamp is accompanied by return of pulsations, which progressively become stronger in a few minutes.

Emboli may occlude the brachial artery at its bifurcation. Pulsations to that point and absence beyond it are associated with a cold, pale hand, causing the patient discomfort. Angiography is informative regarding the distal extent of occlusion of radial and ulnar arteries and of the latter's tributary, the interosseous artery (Fig. 4-33). Local anesthesia permits a longitudinal incision medial to the biceps tendon, a 1-cm transverse component at the antecubital crease, and continuation into the proximal forearm. The brachial artery is mobilized distally to visualize its bifurcation. A transverse incision 1 cm proximal to the bifurcation permits guidance of balloon catheters (4 Fr. Fogarty) into both radial and ulnar branches for simultaneous inflation and withdrawal (Fig. 4-34). Each catheter is reinserted, and alternate inflation of balloons permits estimation of back-bleeding. Unsatisfactory back-bleeding demands further angiography. Not recommended is insertion of deflated catheters for measured distances into the hand, inflation of balloons, and catheter withdrawal, for this has resulted in severe ischemia of fingers, presumably due to fragmentation or manipulation of the thrombus into distal arteries. If hand color and other evidences of circulation are not satisfactory, incisions through the palm to expose palmar arch and digital arteries has restored circulation.

CORONARY ARTERIES

Clinically, there is limited frequency of emboli to coronary arteries. Embolic causes of ischemic symptoms and signs in myocardium in logical candidates may be confirmed subsequently by angiography. Isolated studies of enzymatic lytic treatment and of surgical attempts have been reported. In atherosclerotic lesions, intractable angina without infarction and ischemic electrocardiographic patterns

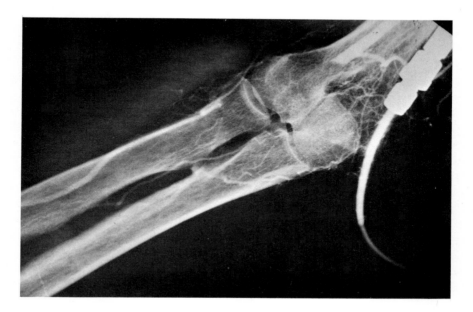

Figure 4-33. BRACHIAL ARTERY EMBOLUS. Opacification of the radial artery is more dense than the ulnar artery. The interosseous artery, which usually takes origin from the ulnar artery, is not filled with contrast medium.

consistent with stenoses or occlusions along the distribution of the right coronary artery may be the most hopeful preangiographic conditions. Discrete stenoses or occlusions in proximal portions of coronary arteries are accessible surgically. Among the best results (survival and function) of direct operation upon coronary arteries were those instances with major obstruction limited to the proximal portion of the right coronary artery and syphilitic occlusions of the ostia of either artery.

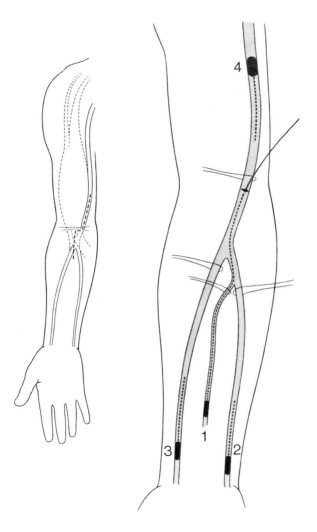

Figure 4-34. EMBOLECTOMY OF ARTERIES OF ARM AND FOREARM. The brachial artery's superficial location permits ready exposure, control, and handling. Its bifurcation and the interosseous artery must be visualized to assure entry with Fogarty catheters for embolectomy, thrombectomy, and certainty of distal patency. The order of entry is indicated numerically. The transverse component of skin incision minimizes the likelihood of contracture. Systemic heparinization is used; 5-0 suture material closes transverse arteriotomy incision.

Until recently, electrocardiographic evidence of diffuse distribution of myocardial ischemia suggested vascular lesions irreparable by conventional techniques. Angiographic confirmation of diffuse distribution of occlusive processes in coronary arteries was considered a contraindication to direct procedures. Since 1967, however, anastomotic procedures to the usually patent distal anterior descending coronary arteries have proved highly successful. Internal mammary arteries or segments of vein interposed between aorta and right and left coronary arteries have delivered 40 to 75 cc increased blood flow per minute per graft. Congestive heart failure may not yield to coronary artery bypass operations, while excision of malfunctioning portions of ventricular wall contributes significantly to hemodynamic improvement. Valve lesions (e.g., aortic stenosis, mitral regurgitation) associated with coronary insufficiency contribute to excess work of the myocardium. Aortic stenosis with angina and gradient greater than 50 mm Hg is a specific indication for correction of valve pathology. The precise interrelation of valve pathology, coronary artery disease, and myocardial hypofunction is yet to be demonstrated. In instances when valve pathology was contained, improvement after repair or replacement of the valve has been attributed to deficient coronary circulation. Conversely poor results after surgery only upon coronary arteries have been attributed to failure to correct the valve abnormality.

Responses to sodium-loading before operation and 14 days postoperative appear to identify patients who have benefited from corrective heart surgery and those who have not. Greater than 60 percent of sodium ingested over a seven-day period is excreted in the urine of patients who are responding favorably. Thus, an unsatisfactory response to correction of only one of several possible causes of cardiac malfunction may be detected early enough to consider performing additional corrective measures, heroic though they may seem. In reality, omission of potentially useful procedures may be radical, not conservative.

MESENTERIC ARTERIES

The history and findings of acute occlusion of the superior mesenteric artery are classic, yet many instances are overlooked. Suspicion of the diagnosis warrants angiography before operation, if angiography can be done expeditiously and well. Atherosclerotic pathology in celiac axis, aorta, or renal arteries may influence the judgment and operative approach of the surgeon. Bypass procedure may be elected rather than local endarterectomy and thrombectomy. It may be possible and advisable to correct chronic pathology of celiac or renal arteries at the time of embolectomy.

Uncertainty of diagnosis of possible ischemia of bowel in the presence of severe coexisting disease fosters delay in operation, yet angiograms rarely are performed. An extensive library of normal vascular patterns of visceral arteries is available to compare with angiograms yet to be performed in quantity upon patients with mesenteric infarction. While overlooked, undiagnosed, and untreated necrosis of bowel portends certain fatality, 85 percent mortality accompanies current modes of operative exploration. Without angiography to spur operation earlier these figures may not improve.

Patients who consistently have crampy upper abdominal pain soon after meals, of an intensity that causes them to eat less and to lose weight, and in whom epigastric bruits exist, must be considered candidates for angiography and arterial reconstruction to relieve ischemia of the splanchnic circulation. When history and examinations exclude other sites and causes of symptoms, and angiography discloses stenoses or occlusions of celiac or superior mesenteric arteries or both, arterial operation is indicated. There may be merely aching or distention, and symptoms may occur more often or less frequently than the patient takes meals. Apparent psychologic cripples with distinct, severe arterial insufficiency should be operated upon. Conversely, patients with stenosis of only one of the visceral arteries, vague variable symptoms, absence of pathology on examination of gall bladder, stomach, intestines, colon, pancreas, and kidneys, and without weight loss pose a relative contraindication. Serious coexisting and unremediable cardiovascular diseases may be absolute contraindications to operation. Technical aspects of surgery are made more difficult when there have been previous multiple celiotomies or when aneurysmal or occlusive processes of the aorta are advanced. Few surgeons have broad experience in this anatomic area, which imposes the greater likelihood of failing to achieve revascularization expeditiously. A modest amount of time in the morgue familiarizes one with details of exposure, routes for tunnels for prostheses, and sites of arteriotomies to achieve satisfactory reconstruction of visceral circulation.

RENAL ARTERIES

Rarely is renal artery embolus diagnosed. The acute angle of emergence of renal arteries from the aorta favoring entrapment of emboli often is unappreciated by physicians. Sudden oliguria in a patient prone to embolization demands angiography. Occlusion of a single renal artery in a patient seriously ill with heart disease may seem to contraindicate abdominal aortic exploration. Physicians may doom both kidney and patient with the poorly founded concern that contrast medium may contribute to renal injury. Established diagnosis is needed to force decision and appropriate action. The same patient may need and survive corrective heart surgery concurrently with renal artery operation; either procedure alone may be unreasonable without correcting function of both heart and kidney.

Experience with renal artery embolectomy is too limited for authoritative comment concerning absolute and relative indications for embolectomy, although it seems tenable to conclude that any patient with demonstrated bilateral renal artery occlusion has scant possibility to survive. Prompt restoration of renal blood flow, supportive measures, and dialysis as indicated, may be compatible with survival. Recorded long-term consequences of untreated unilateral renal artery occlusion, while limited, permit the inference of double jeopardy; function of one kidney is lost, and the second is jeopardized by the initiation of a serious new disease. We have seen three cases of acute renal artery occlusions treated without operation that demonstrated early onset of hypertension accompanied by high renin levels in renal venous blood, relieved in every instance by nephrectomy (Fig. 4-35). It would have been better to have restored the circulation early enough for survival of both kidneys.

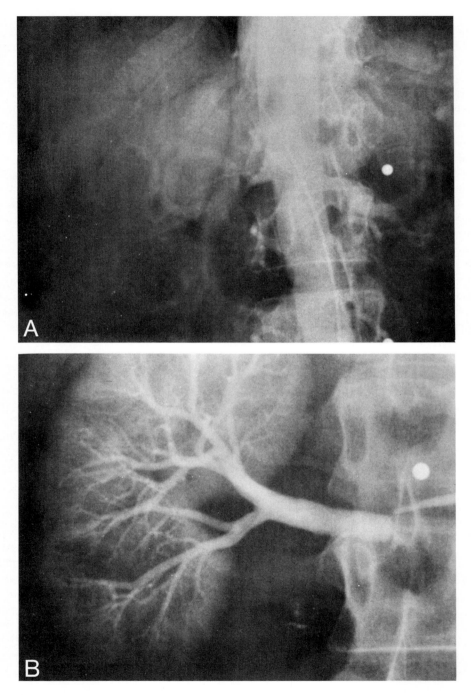

Figure 4-35. SELECTIVE RENAL ANGIOGRAPHY. (A) Aortogram in hypertensive patient discloses apparent occlusion of right renal artery. (B) Selective renal angiogram (? "sheath" or intramural injection) was followed by pain, hematuria, arterial thrombosis, and renal infarction requiring nephrectomy.

Stenosis of one or both renal arteries from atherosclerosis, associated with recent onset of hypertension, and evidence of decreased renal function coincident with the arterial lesion suggest that restoration of lumen caliber will restore function and relieve hypertension. Elevation of renin concentration in venous blood from a kidney with arterial stenosis strengthens the indication for operation. Kidney dysfunction bordering on uremia may make operation the acceptable alternative to death.

Patients with symptomatic generalized occlusive vascular disease may have systolic hypertension and borderline diastolic hypertension, interpreted clinically as consequences of rigidity in the aorta and decreased capacity of distribution of stroke volume through major arteries. Abdominal bruits may be caused by stenoses in renal arteries as well as in the aorta, both evident on angiography. It is known that renin concentrations decline spontaneously in long-standing hypertension. Indications for operation appear less well-founded in these circumstances. If surgical correction of aorta-iliac stenosis is performed, renal artery lesions should be corrected. Renal artery reconstruction may be done even though femoropopliteal sclerosis is so advanced that aorta-iliac and distal reconstructions are contraindicated.

RENAL ARTERY ENDARTERECTOMY. Renal artery endarterectomy is performed through midline or subcostal incisions. Patients' spines need not be hyperextended. Mannitol infusions are used as originally advocated by Barry—1 gram (5 cc) of a 20 percent solution per minute for 30 minutes, followed by 1 cc per minute of a 5 percent solution. Upon release of occluding clamps on the renal artery, 12.5 grams is infused as a bolus, a modification used by Poutasse. Using hydration and mannitol, bilateral renal artery occlusion uniformly has been well tolerated for periods of one hour at normal body temperature.

Incision in the posterior parietal peritoneum medial to the inferior mesenteric vein and dissection along the aorta to the left renal vein fail to make renal arteries accessible until additional landmarks are visualized. The left renal vein is cleared of tissue on to the first centimeter of the inferior vena cava both below and above the vein. The right renal vein is not visualized. Left adrenal and spermatic or ovarian veins are ligated and divided. Tissue is readily separated from the aorta, the superior mesenteric artery, and both renal arteries. Almost invariably the right renal artery is higher, and commonly the left renal artery appears kinked at its point of emergence due to left posterior rotation of the aorta. Tangential clamping permits endarterectomy of the origins of the renal arteries separately. Transverse clamping of the aorta and the superior mesenteric artery and simultaneous exposure of the origins of both renal arteries by transverse aortotomy extended onto renal arteries may be done (Fig. 4-36). Plaques of the aortic wall that intrude upon the orifices of the renal arteries but extend only a few millimeters into the renal arteries may be removed by longitudinal aortotomy. Visibility into the renal artery lumen assures leaving nonthrombogenic lining of each renal artery. This appears an especially desirable technique when multiple renal artery kinks or occlusions require patch enlargement to relieve them. Incision along its caudal aspect, extending along the lateral aortic wall,

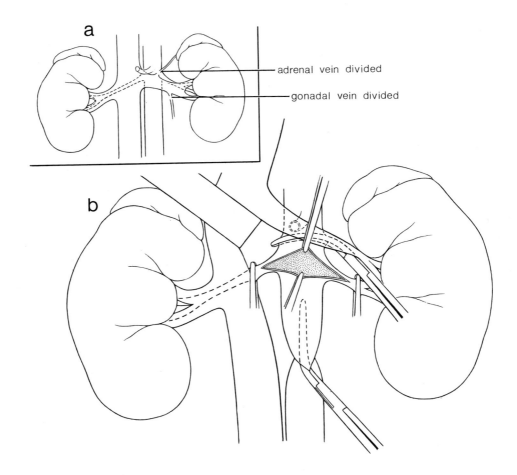

adrenal vein divided

gonadal vein divided

Figure 4-36. RENAL ARTERY ENDARTERECTOMY VIA TRANSVERSE AOR-
TOTOMY. Midline abdominal incision to costal arch at left of xiphoid. Retroperitoneal
exposure medial to inferior mesenteric vein. Division of left adrenal and gonadal veins
(a) permits extensive mobilization of left renal vein for operative access to junction of
aorta with renal arteries, and suprarenal control of aorta. Transverse aortotomy carried
into both renal arteries facilitates removal of thick plaque of aorta extending into renal
arteries (b). Left renal vein is cephalad and anterior to suprarenal aortic clamp. Infrarenal clamp occludes lumbar arteries also.

accommodates a diamond-shaped patch, and has been used satisfactorily more
often than a composite graft into a transverse aortotomy (Fig. 4-37).

It is considered a delusive practice to attempt to define indication for
reconstruction of the renal artery by measurement of pressure gradient or by
calibration of renal artery orifice size with a clamp passed through the aortotomy
site into renal arteries. It is believed decisions should be made by angiography
prior to operation. Attempts at assessment of presence or absence of significant
lesion and degree of imposed stenoses are difficult and misleading. Deliberate

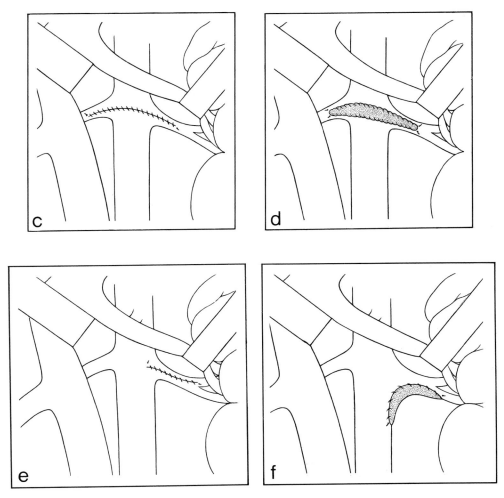

Figure 4-37. RENAL ARTERY ENDARTERECTOMY. Primary and prosthetic patch closures of transverse aortotomy (c, d). Renal artery must not be narrowed. Patch closure depicts separate suture on each side of patch, *not* tied to each other. Cephalad aortic clamp may have been placed obliquely, below right and above left renal arteries (e). Not uncommonly the left renal artery origin is displaced posteriorly. Incision along axis of renal artery may continue onto aorta to facilitate endarterectomy of its orifice and to relieve a kink effect. A patch may be necessary to enlarge primary and branch artery orifices (f).

visualization and endarterectomy through a local incision remove doubt (Figs. 4-38 and 4-39). Callow[40] has correlated intrarenal resistance from measurements of flow and pressure with estimation of relief of hypertension by surgical procedures.

    Bypass grafts from distal aorta, iliac artery, and portions of synthetic grafts have been sutured to sides of renal arteries distal to stenoses when diffuse enlargement of the suprarenal aorta has discouraged dissection and clamping of the aorta (see Fig. 3-6, p. 44).

Figure 4-38. RENAL ARTERY ENDARTERECTOMY AND AORTIC RECON-
STRUCTION. Sites of clamping and of incisions are shown (a). Adequate caliber of
aorta and minimal extension of plaque into renal arteries allows good visualization of
first few millimeters of *insides* of renal arteries, as aorta-renal artery junction is retracted
laterally (b). The distal end of the plaque may be incised, *never* avulsed.

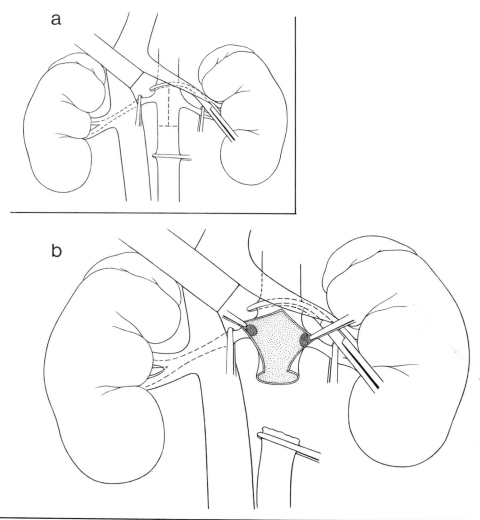

Figure 4-39. Short incision in axis of renal artery permits precise incisional termination
of endarterectomy and assures free flow of blood across nonthrombogenic site (d, e).
Left renal arteriotomy incision closed, and aortotomy closure carried distal to renal
arteries to permit restoration of flow through renal arteries (f). Vertical application of
clamp has two purposes—facility, and intent to have teeth of clamp cushioned by aortic
wall, precluding clamp trauma to suture material.

Primary and prosthetic patch closure techniques of aorta (g, h). Again, note
separate sutures each side of patch, *not* tied to each other. Continuity of aorta would be
restored through end-to-end (preferred) or end-to-side grafts to distal arteries. The aortic
stump distal to the excised segment of infrarenal aorta (Fig. 4-38, b) is closed with
continuous suture prior to anastomosis of prosthetic graft to the reconstructed proximal
aorta.

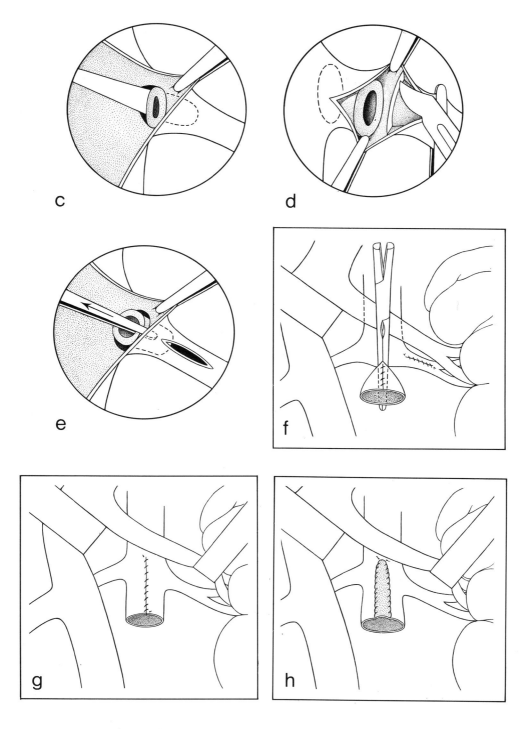

Figure 4-39.   RENAL ARTERY ENDARTERECTOMY

Fibromuscular hyperplasia of renal arteries has been treated by excision and substitution with saphenous vein graft, and by patch (composite grafts carried onto branch arteries). Transverse incision from the sacrospinal muscles posteriorly to the lateral border of the rectus muscles anteriorly provides ready access to retroperitoneal structures and easy development of the operative field, including retraction of viscera and isolation of the renal and common iliac arteries. Proximally, the renal artery is dissected until hyperplasia is palpable, and a site is selected for later ligation in continuity or for division. Two or three branches of the renal artery are isolated distally, assuring identification by comparison with angiographic findings (Fig. 4-40). Depending upon the caliber of the distal renal artery, a graft of woven dacron 6 or 8 mm internal diameter is selected. The graft need not be preclotted prior to systemic administration of heparin. Anastomosis to the iliac artery is accomplished first, where bevelling of the graft is not necessary. Not uncommonly, operative enlargement of the lumen must extend into a subdivision of the renal artery. Here, precise tailoring to conform with considerations for laminar flow to the renal artery will assure optimum function. Sutures of 5-0 tycron, tevdek, or polyethylene are used. Closure must be performed with ideal exposure. Closure of arteriotomy over a catheter may be cumbersome, and stretched artery or graft may constrict upon removal of stent, as unsatisfactory clinical course and angiogram may confirm. A small-bore polyethylene catheter on gentle suction (50 mm Hg) lying in the opened artery can provide perfect visibility for reconstruction. When a composite vein graft is being sutured into the end of an arteriotomy in a small vessel, interrupted sutures near the ends will minimize any likelihood of constriction.

BYPASS GRAFT FOR CORRECTION OF FIBROMUSCULAR HYPERPLASIA.   Logic permits the conclusion that prosthetic bypass graft is an acceptable, if not the preferable, procedure to increase blood flow to the kidney. The large requirement of blood flow through a kidney obligates high flow rate through a graft, virtually assuring early and long-term patency. Precise attention to technical details of anastomosis minimizes thrombogenic conditions. The advantages of minimum dissection in the local area and the assurance of optimal size and strength of graft material allow a brief operation.

Prosthetic grafts for renal revascularization have been advocated for years. The presumed superiority of autogenous saphenous veins made the use of veins our first choice. Subsequently the proximity of the ovarian vein led to its use twice, and disruption both times precipitated resort to prostheses to minimize the time of renal ischemia by clamping superimposed upon the hypovolemic and hypotensive state. In reviewing the possible advantages of prostheses in overcoming stenosis of the renal artery, we recalled that we had used prosthetic grafts satisfactorily when diffuse dilatation of the infradiaphragmatic aorta cast doubt upon the wisdom of dissection or clamping of that hypertensive aorta and in instances of total replacement of the abdominal aorta.

AORTA-ILIAC BIFURCATION

EMBOLI.   Embolic occlusion of the aortic bifurcation usually causes serious ischemic symptoms in thighs, legs, and feet. Sudden onset of pain, coldness, numb-

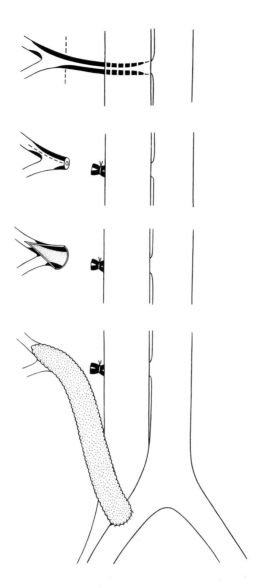

Figure 4-40. FIBROMUSCULAR HYPER-
PLASIA OF RENAL ARTERY. Reasoning
that large flows through short segments
favor long-term patency of prosthetic grafts,
a better operation easier to perform in less
time is advocated. Angiograms which disclose
the site and extent of stenosis permit precise preoperative planning. The graft is
anastomosed to the iliac artery before the
renal artery, to minimize ischemic time. (See
Figure 4-11, p. 70, for details of anastomosis of bevelled graft.)

ness, pallor, and paresis are alarming to patient and physician. Vessels are pulse-less distal to mid-abdomen. Symptoms are more severe when thrombus propagates distally, or when "showers" of emboli also occlude smaller peripheral arteries. The certainty of distal embolization may not be apparent until operation or angiography; spontaneous fragmentation and dislodgement of saddle embolus may occur, obstructing arteries of limbs. Pain, pallor, and paralysis may become worse in distal portions of limbs. Improvement in color in proximal limbs may mean relief of vasospasm without movement of embolus. Pathologic ischemia may cause this due to neural dysfunction; lessened symptoms need not imply improvement.

Patients who are debilitated or dying from other causes or those with severe heart failure may seem too ill for any operation. Occasionally, patients in this category survive with viable limbs without operative relief of arterial obstruction. Thrombolytic agents (urokinase and streptokinase) have been known to yield complete relief of bilateral obstruction of major arteries in hours or days.

EMBOLECTOMY OF ABDOMINAL AORTIC BIFURCATION.   Operation soon after onset of symptoms, without angiography, is indicated for embolic obstruction of the aortic bifurcation. If heparin has been given, spinal anesthesia is contraindicated, to avoid the risk of hematoma around or into the spinal cord. Patients may be too uncomfortable to be manipulated for spinal anesthesia despite its theoretical advantages over general anesthesia in relieving vasospasm. Anticoagulation is continued throughout the operation. Femoral triangles are always included in the area prepared for operation. At laparotomy, gentle palpation at the bifurcation of the common iliac arteries discloses whether embolic material has reached that level. Usually embolus is confined to proximal portions of common iliac arteries, and protrudes more prominently into one. Encircling tapes are placed on external iliac arteries distal to the palpable embolus, and noncrushing clamps are applied to these arteries. Without encircling dissection of the aorta, a vascular occlusive clamp is applied to the aorta. Incision is made longitudinally into the antero-lateral aspect of the proximal portion of the common iliac artery containing more of the embolus. The embolus extrudes itself or may be plucked from the vessel. Pressure ("milking") with fingers, probing with open-ended suction tip or catheter, and transient release and reapplication of proximal aortic clamp, then distal clamps, assures delivery of all local embolic and thrombotic material, and the amount of back-bleeding gives a useful indication of patency of distal vessels.

If an embolus is at the bifurcation of an iliac artery, distal control of branches and an incision opposite the orifice of the hypogastric artery permit removal of the embolus and evaluation and instrumentation of the internal iliac artery. If there is uncertainty about the completeness of the removal of the thrombus and embolus from the contralateral iliac artery, the original incision in the proximal wall of the common iliac artery may be extended onto the aorta or a second incision made in the opposite iliac artery. It is purposeful to make incisions that are near bifurcations of arteries 120 to 180 degrees from the branch. This permits ease of manipulation half-way around the circumference of a mass lesion in the lumen or the wall of an artery, improving visibility of the object being dissected. This provides visual perspective for the preservation of integrity of the orifice during dissection and manipulation at that site and during closure of the arteriotomy. Incisions into walls of both arteries near a bifurcation should be as widely separated as consistent with surgical ease to avoid problems inherent in reconstruction of a Y-shaped incision. Restoration of pulses of good quality in hypogastric arteries and at femoral arteries justifies closure of the abdominal incision.

Control of iliac arteries and aorta assures confinement of fragments and complete removal of embolus and thrombus, the least likelihood of blood loss and technical complications, and immediate complete restoration of normal circulation in vessels proximal to the inguinal ligament.

Retrograde use of catheters via femoral arteries to aspirate or extract embolus and thrombus may be used if risk of general anesthesia and laparotomy seems prohibitive. Formidable technical problems may be encouraged and created as catheters are passed through atherosclerotic stenosed vessels. During withdrawal of the catheter, as the embolus is compressed against the bifurcation of the iliac artery, it is all but inevitable that material will obstruct the hypogastric arteries. Dislodgement of plaques and disruption of the arterial wall can occur when emboli do not fragment into particles small enough to pass through an external artery. Thrombus adherent to walls may not be removed, leaving thrombogenic surfaces. The many reports of successful use of femoral artery routes of embolectomy of aortic bifurcation do not endorse it as a preferred technique.

EMBOLECTOMY IN LARGE TRIBUTARY ARTERIES.   The presence of pulses in a lower extremity does not exclude the possibility of embolic occlusion of hypogastric or profunda femoris or peroneal arteries (Fig. 4-41). Embolic obstruction at those sites may occur spontaneously or secondary to blind manipulation as with balloon catheters. Young patients with arteries highly remediable because they are supple, with smooth intima and adequate lumina, pose interesting dilemmas when emboli occur. Collateral circulation may be adequate for limb survival, but future circulation and function may be compromised by further emboli. This problem seems especially perplexing following corrective heart surgery, when prosthetic valve sites which initiate emboli may be anticipated to threaten recurrences indefinitely. It is mandatory to achieve adequate anticoagulation at once, and it is desirable to remove the emboli. Emboli in patients with coronary or rheumatic heart disease who have not had heart operations need to have the two problems considered separately. Treat the emboli as though the cause did not exist. Give careful consideration to the virtues of physiologic study (e.g., cardiac catheterization, coronary angiography) upon which to base decision for anticoagulation or operation upon the heart.

ANEURYSMS.   The detection in the abdominal aorta of an aneurysm that is symptomatic (e.g., pain in the back or inguinal regions), expanding, or greater than 7 cm in diameter is an indication for resection and replacement. Advanced age or severe associated diseases may be contraindications to operation when symptoms are minimal and the size of the mass is stable. Operation upon aneurysms in patients with recent coronary artery insufficiency may be deferred until

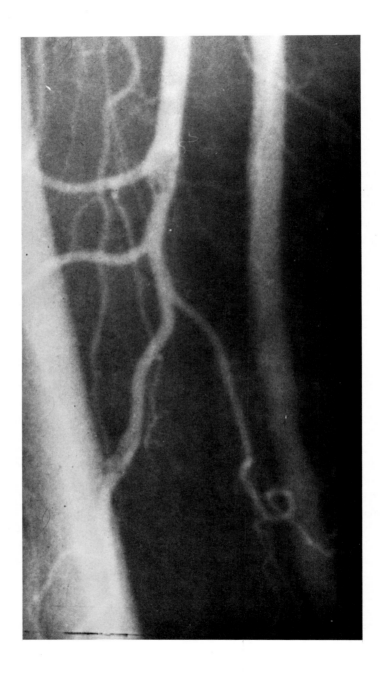

Figure 4-41. UNSUSPECTED EMBOLUS. This angiogram portrays a dividend of routine angiography in the "search and correct" concept of treatment of emboli. A below-knee incision sufficed for removal of symptomatic distal emboli. *Only* awareness of this lesion compelled femoral arteriotomy.

myocardial stability occurs. Suprarenal aneurysm increases operative risk considerably. Aneurysms in iliac arteries may coexist and not uncommonly are sites of rupture.

STENOSIS AND OCCLUSION. Prenecrotic and necrotic lesions of toes and feet secondary to obstructive processes in the aorta and its branches demand reversal by arterial reconstruction if that is possible technically and physiologically. Rest pain seriously portends ischemic necrosis. There is indication for restorative vascular surgery when gainful employment or enjoyable existence is limited by symptoms. Operative restitution of mainline flow may be a luxury if symptoms and disability are mild and compatible with useful living. Operation may be unwarranted when the probability of successful outcome is dubious, or when the disability of conservative therapy or amputation may be borne by an inactive octogenarian or coped with by a younger, well-motivated person. Preventive arterial reconstruction is practiced far more commonly than this is admitted or advocated. For example, many sites of stenoses of varying degree are corrected when aorta-iliac endarterectomy is performed. Experience has shown unsatisfactory results of incomplete correction of lesions. Thus, maneuvers continue until adequate in-flow and run-off are secured in a given area. Employment of this concept is espoused in relief of renal artery stenoses combined with reconstruction or replacement of the abdominal aorta (Fig. 4-42).

ILIAC ARTERIES. "Iliac equivalent" disease is a term referring to marked limitation of flow to an extremity, due to reduced volume of flow and pressure from single, tandem, or multiple obstructing processes in the iliac artery and distally (see pp. 16 and 130). Marked diminution or absence of pulse at the groin suggests iliac luminal pathology which limits flow and pressure to the periphery. Near-normal femoral pulse and pressure may mask the same degree of iliac narrowing as when a high resistance obstruction exists in the femoral artery a short distance distally. The descriptions and classifications of Wesolowski,[53] Haimovici,[62] Imparato,[50] and Strandness[70] attempt to explain the phenomena, but a straightforward clinical or laboratory test differentiating mechanisms and degrees of iliac stenosis remains to be developed. A suggested workable plan is the following:

In patients well enough to tolerate the operation, restore aorta-iliac or aorta-femoral continuity when complaints and angiographic findings demand this. Observe and record blood flow and pressure before and after reconstruction to demonstrate what is commonly seen—blood flow tripled, from a prereconstruction mean flow of 100 rising to 300 to 500 ml per min. The commonly practiced alternative, a "see what happens" attitude, may be successful ("right for the wrong reason"). Failure may force an additional procedure, conventional or extended. Axillo-femoral and cross-over grafts have virtues and drawbacks; they cannot deliver as much flow as aorta-iliac or aorta-femoral reconstruction, nor will they remain patent as long.

BIFURCATION ENDARTERECTOMY. The classic approach to aorta-iliac endarterectomy is through two arterial incisions. The major incision crosses the junction of parent (aorta) and one tributary (iliac) artery. The second incision is confined to the other tributary, approaching and even crossing the junction, but not joining the major incision. The distal extent of both the major and secondary incisions permits precise termination of intravascular dissection, so that blood will flow across smooth vessel lining. The essence of endarterectomy—access to the entire obstructive process—is preserved. Retrograde operation through the second incision frees the plaque from the bifurcation carina with a certainty that is not possible through a single incision.

Hypogastric artery stenoses at origins occur frequently. Multiple plaques intrude upon the cross-sectional area of proximal portions of branches of the hypogastric artery. Operation is often unsuccessful in improving blood flow and

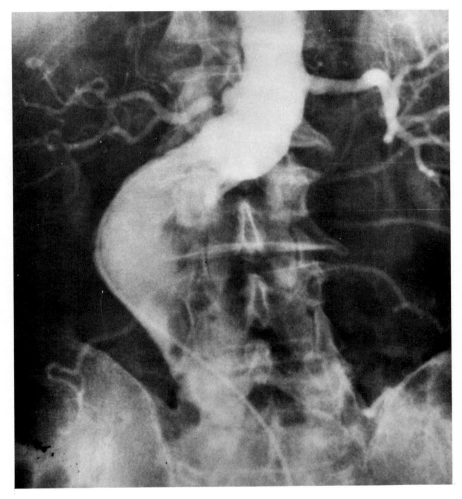

Figure 4-42. DIVIDEND OF "ROUTINE" ANGIOGRAPHY. Preoperative routine angiography disclosed significant stenosis of right renal artery, readily relieved at aneurysmectomy. Fortunate site of origin permitted aortic clamping distal to left renal artery.

thus is not only rarely indicated but frequently contraindicated. Promoting even limited flow through diseased hypogastric arteries may be effected most readily by not disturbing arterial plaques. Iliac endarterectomy may be terminated proximal to the origin of the hypogastric artery. The distal end of the common iliac artery may be closed, and a bypass graft inserted into the external iliac or common femoral artery. Marked relief of peripheral symptoms generally follows operative restoration of iliac flow. Edwards[49] has advocated operation forthwith, without angiography, reasoning from experience that if there is structural integrity of the limb, the profunda femoris arteries must be open. However, Wylie[54] advocates operation cephalad of the inguinal ligament to minimize complication of groin wounds (e.g., infection, flexion of graft, lymph fistula). The frequency of stenosis of the origins of profunda femoris arteries permits and encourages selectivity of procedure for greatest benefits and least risk of complication when angiography guides the choice of procedure. Operation distal to the inguinal ligament, restoring the caliber of the profunda femoris artery when indicated, may be necessary for optimal distal blood flow. Blaisdell's extensive and favorable experience with bypass grafts supports this view.[48]

Virtual absence of lumina in highly sclerotic femoral artery distribution and distal arteries may predict the failure of aorta-iliac and aorta-femoral reconstructive procedures. Avoidance of any operation may be preferable to risking or hastening amputation which may not heal except at proximal thigh level.

AORTA-DISTAL EXTERNAL ILIAC BYPASS. Spontaneous and recurrent atherosclerotic occlusions of the proximal 3 cm of external iliac arteries may have special clinical significance which has been overlooked. Recurrent ischemic symptoms, diminished pulses, and demonstrable stenoses soon after aorta-iliac endarterectomy have led to closer examination of this site in angiograms and at operations. Although concentric atherosclerotic lesions of iliac arteries may appear to end at the orifices of the hypogastric and external iliac arteries, often they continue into the latter. The diameter of the proximal 1 to 4 cm of external iliac arteries, compared with the succeeding segment, is constricted by one-third in many patients. Palpation and inspection of this area before and after longitudinal incision discloses firm, thick, fibrous wall and unyielding lumen size. The intima may appear nonsclerotic, yet it fragments and separates with attempts at intraluminal dilatation. Microscopic examination of tissue from this region discloses no evidence of fibromuscular hyperplasia. Suggested treatment is patch angioplasty (composite reconstruction) or aorta-external iliac bypass graft (Fig. 4-43). Two aspects of the latter have seemed especially logical and practical—placing arteriotomies on the anteromedial aspect of external iliac arteries immediately proximal to the inguinal ligaments, and end-to-end anastomosis of the aorta with the graft. The end-to-end aorta-graft anastomosis favors laminar flow and obligates all blood to pass through the graft, yielding increased patency rates. With the handles of the clamps on the medial side of the vessel, their application compressing the atherosclerotic plaques of the dorsal walls of the iliac arteries in an anteroposterior plane least disturbs them or their attachments to media. Simultaneously, rotation of the clamps elevates the medial aspect of the artery for incision and anastomosis. The anteromedial locations of the limbs of the graft ensure the least tendency of

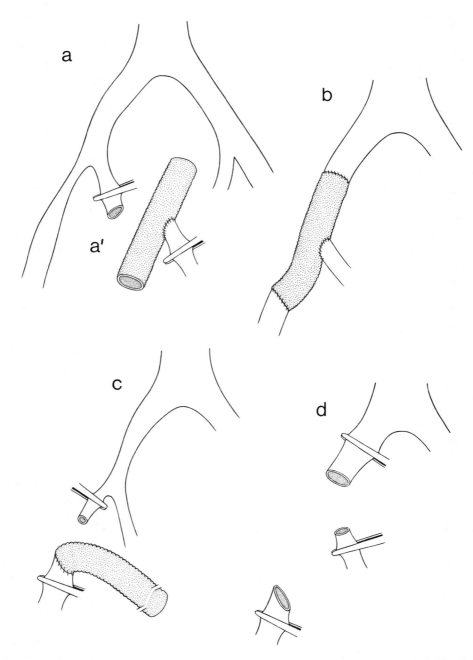

Figure 4-43. ARTERIAL RECONSTRUCTION AT BIFURCATIONS. If excision of bifurcation is necessary, it may not be necessary to interrupt all three vessels at once (d). The smaller caliber (and frequent heavy plaques) of hypogastric artery (a) or a bevelled anastomosis of external iliac artery (c) may require a longer time for meticulous suturing. Physiologic and technical benefits of maintenance of some circulation while one of those anastomoses is performed may be achieved employing maneuvers illustrated in a, a', and c.

rotation, since circumstances of gravity and anatomy in the supine patient favor the course of the graft on the medial rather than anterior aspects of iliac arteries.

The technical considerations just described are intended to *contradict those diagrams appearing in certain atlases of surgical procedures* which illustrate insertion of limbs of bypass grafts into the lateral aspect of distal iliac arteries. Rarely do circumstances favor such sites of insertion. Some illustrations of artery incisions and graft anastomoses into the anteromedial aspect of internal iliac arteries have depicted lateral locations of the handles of clamps, the effect restricting mobilization of the operative site, to the disadvantage of the surgeon.

Bypass graft from the aorta to the distal external iliac artery is recommended for its advantages of least duration of interruption of circulation, provision of a conduit of known uniform caliber, strength, and durability, and avoidance of technical problems and complications inherent in aorta-iliac endarterectomy. End-to-end anastomosis of the aorta to the proximal portion of the bifurcation graft obligates implantation of limbs into the sides of iliac arteries to provide retrograde flow to pelvic vessels. Theoretical disadvantages of missing an opportunity to enlarge the orifices of hypogastric arteries are relative. The impracticability and incidence of thrombosis following attempts at endarterectomy of hypogastric arteries have already been cited (see p. 117). Doubtless, more occlusions of hypogastric arteries have been caused by operation than have been relieved by such procedures. Acceptable compensation in principle is inherent in the delivery of the large volume and pressure of blood from bypass grafts to circumflex iliac and external pudendal arteries originating from distal external iliac arteries.

The decision to insert grafts into external iliac arteries rather than into common femoral arteries must be supported by angiographic certainty that there is no need to enlarge the lumina of common or profunda femoris arteries. Theoretical advantages of avoiding incisions in proximal thighs and crossing sites of flexion by vascular grafts must not be compromised by limitations of blood flow through highly stenotic distal arteries. Preoperative estimations should be challenged by blood flow measurements and angiograms during operation.

AORTA-FEMORAL RECONSTRUCTION. Endarterectomy of more than the proximal few centimeters of the external iliac artery is not performed. Blind endarterectomy with strippers may not enjoy the high rate of success as does a bypass graft from the aorta to common femoral arteries. End-to-end anastomosis of the aorta to the bifurcation graft restores optimal flow characteristics. It is likely that end-to-end anastomosis of the limbs of the graft to the ends of common femoral arteries would have the same salubrious effect, but it has seemed advisable not to deprive the pelvic iliac arteries of major blood flow. Thus, bevelled ends of the limbs of grafts are anastomosed to the sides of common femoral arteries. Incisions to receive aorta-femoral grafts may be made opposite the orifices of profunda femoris arteries to permit endarterectomy of the latter if necessary, or in continuity with the proximal centimeter of the profunda femoris artery.

The operative procedure exposes the retroperitoneal aorta and iliac arteries. If the extent and severity (thickness) of atheromatous plaques are confined

to abdominal vessels, aorta-iliac endarterectomy is performed. Commonly, hypogastric and external iliac arteries are sclerotic to an extent greater than estimated
from angiograms, and common femoral arteries are elected as the distal extent of
reconstruction (Fig. 4-44). These arteries are isolated, and retroperitoneal tunnels
created by blunt dissection along iliac arteries, anterior to ureters, communicate
with the principal operative area. Woven graft material is used in preference to
knitted, to minimize blood loss. Preclotting is not necessary in woven grafts but
is essential in knitted grafts. The limbs of the bifurcation graft, usually 8 or 9.5
mm inside diameter, are drawn from the abdomen into the femoral wounds, and
held with hemostatic clamps to prevent rotation. Heparin is administered intravenously.

The physiologic practicability and the logic of performing distal anastomoses first limits the period of deprivation of blood to the limbs to no more
than 30 minutes at a time. Vascular clamps with broad blades are applied to the

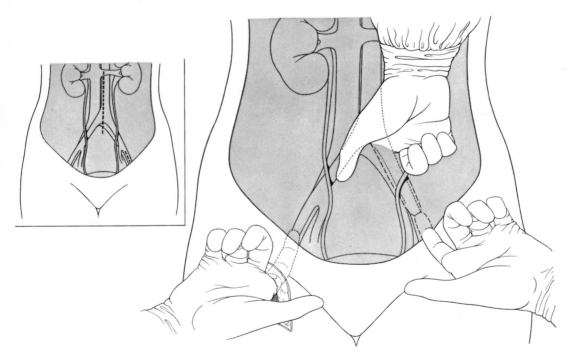

Figure 4-44. RETROPERITONEAL TUNNELS FOR BYPASS GRAFTS. Blunt dissection retroperitoneally along courses of iliac arteries displaces ureters ventrally. The
proximal retroperitoneal incision allows introduction of finger at level of aortic bifurcation. On the left, the opposing finger enters the retroperitoneum over the external
iliac artery proximal to the inguinal ligament. On the right, incision over the femoral
triangle permits finger dissection along sheath of common femoral and external iliac
arteries, beneath inguinal ligament. A long Kelly clamp passed proximally in each tunnel
grasps folded-over ends of limbs of graft, delivering each limb into distal operative
wounds. Appropriate stretch and tension are determined at that time, and clamps are
placed on limbs of graft to locate sites for bevelled transection and to maintain appropriate alignment of graft.

common, deep, and superficial femoral arteries; arteriotomy is made, and the bevelled limb of the graft is sutured to the artery. A hemostatic clamp is applied to the graft 1 cm from the anastomosis, and clamps are removed from femoral artery segments. The second side is treated similarly.

The aorta is clamped to permit division and closure of the distal end 2 cm above the inferior mesenteric artery. The proximal clamp lies between the renal and the inferior mesenteric arteries; the latter transiently is occluded separately. Endarterectomy of the infrarenal segment may be performed, and a single layer anastomosis of the aorta to the graft is made with continuous 3-0 suture material. Just prior to completion of the anastomosis, the graft is allowed to back-bleed freely. Clamps are removed permanently from femoral limbs for this, then a Kelly clamp is applied to the aortic portion of the graft while the anastomosis is completed. The Kelly and aortic clamps are removed.

It is important to prevent clotting during the reconstruction. Assuming there is hemostasis during isolation of the vessels, little bleeding is expected after 75 mg of heparin is administered. Additional doses of 50 mg of heparin are given every 60 minutes until the clamps are released and flow is restored to both lower extremities. Protamine sulfate is given intravenously as the clamps are released, in dosage equal to the total amount of heparin given.

CROSS-OVER GRAFTS. Cross-over grafts afford the desiderata of relatively short vascular bridges from sites of good inflow to beds of adequate run-off, possibly invoking advantages of increased velocity of circulation through vessels to the primary extremity. The quantity of blood diverted from the original extremity is incompletely documented, but it appears to cause no undesirable physiologic consequences.

Unilateral iliac artery obstruction appears the principal indication for cross-over grafts. Relative indications are: significant systemic physiologic impairment and estimated unacceptable operative risk to life in the plan to salvage an extremity; anticipated impediments at reoperative site of previously placed bifurcation graft; and alternative to axillo-femoral bypass.

Autogenous, allograft and prosthetic graft materials may be used. The latter appear least applicable for distal anastomosis to small vessels but ideal for femoral-femoral crossover. Fresh or recently obtained long-segment venous allografts permit traversing long distances through subcutaneous tunnels. Operative time and trauma are minimized, and cross-over femoral–below-knee anastomoses may be effected through three "keyhole" incisions. Thus, great benefits accrue in brief periods of physiologic disturbance.

Incisions to originate the cross-over graft should be parallel to the inguinal ligament and should not cross the skin fold between thigh and lower abdomen (Fig. 4-45). The inguinal creases in obese and aged patients commonly lie several inches distal to the inguinal ligament. Accordingly, oblique lower abdominal skin incisions may be made to lie over the femoral triangle, facilitating exposure of the common femoral artery and enhancing healing in an exposed, nonmacerating location.

The incision on the second side may be distal to the inguinal crease parallel to the femoral arteries. The subcutaneous tunnel across the lower abdominal fascia may be joined with the tunnel initiated from the second side (Fig. 4-46). The latter tunnel intentionally is placed lateral to the mass of inguinal lymph nodes. Instrument (Kelly or sponge clamp) or finger dissection or sigmoidoscope may be used to create the tunnel and assure its adequate size. It is important and easy to prevent kinking the graft as it is passed through the tunnel.

The arteriotomy incision is placed on the anteromedial aspect of the common femoral artery. If extensive thick plaque of the dorsal wall of the artery does not contraindicate or preclude vertical application of clamps, 90 degree lateral rotation of them places the anastomotic site in full view of the operator and his assistant. A window or button excision of arterial wall readily accommodates a nonbevelled end of graft. Application of a clamp on the graft 1 cm from the anastomosis permits restoration of flow through the femoral artery.

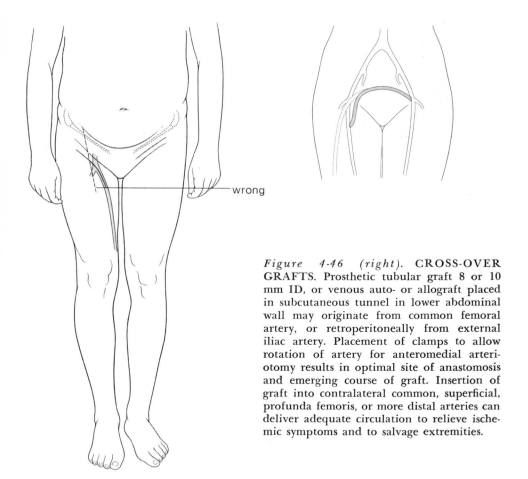

wrong

Figure 4-46 (right). CROSS-OVER GRAFTS. Prosthetic tubular graft 8 or 10 mm ID, or venous auto- or allograft placed in subcutaneous tunnel in lower abdominal wall may originate from common femoral artery, or retroperitoneally from external iliac artery. Placement of clamps to allow rotation of artery for anteromedial arteriotomy results in optimal site of anastomosis and emerging course of graft. Insertion of graft into contralateral common, superficial, profunda femoris, or more distal arteries can deliver adequate circulation to relieve ischemic symptoms and to salvage extremities.

Figure 4-45 (left). EXPOSURE OF CONTENTS OF FEMORAL TRIANGLE. An oblique incision away from inguinal skin crease and fold is preferred to a longitudinal incision which crosses them. In elderly obese patients incision in the abdominal skin (solid line) gives ready access to common femoral artery, and obviates complications of poor healing in a macerated area.

When cross-over graft is a primary procedure, its site of insertion is dictated by angiographic evidence and surgeon's preference (Fig. 4-47). If an arterial operation previously had been performed in the femoral triangle, the difficulties and hazards of local reoperation may be avoided by graft implant into superficial or profunda femoris arteries several centimeters distal to the femoral artery bifurcation.

Long grafts traversing the thigh through blindly constructed tunnels usually require a midthigh incision, which should be several centimeters from the

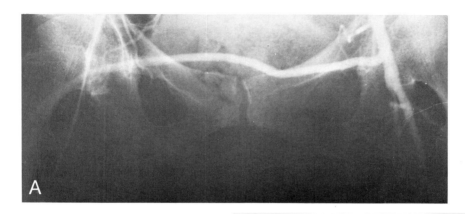

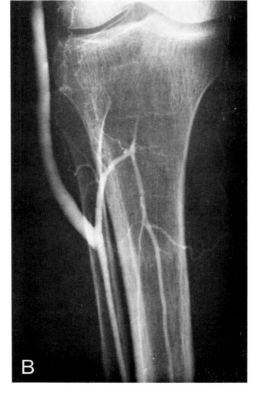

Figure 4-47. CROSS-OVER GRAFT. Allograft saphenous vein from left common femoral artery (A) cross-over to right anterior tibial artery (B).

pathway of the graft. The more dorsal location of this incision, either medial or lateral, allows dependent drainage of serum from the tunnel while minimizing the likelihood of providing an entrance and pathway for infection.

Blood is allowed to flow into the graft to test its integrity, to gauge its length and site of transection, and to assume a "natural" position prior to distal anastomosis. Palpation of distal pulses, noncannulating flow meter measurements, and angiography at operation or within a few days certify achievement of goals of adequate, uncomplicated provision of enhanced perfusion to an ischemic extremity. Perfusion responses to exercise, measured plethysmographically, further attest to the success of cross-over grafts.

Hemostasis should be so secure that drainage is not required. Patients may be helped out of bed the day after operation. It seems advisable to have patients stand, walk, or lie down, deferring sitting for several weeks. Increased tissue tension induced by the edema of operative trauma may threaten luminal patency of grafts if compounded by flexion for periods longer than required to leave or enter bed, to walk, and to sit at stool. At two or three weeks postoperative, with overlying tissues supple, all positions and activity may be allowed.

FEMORAL ARTERIES

ANEURYSMS. Sacciform aneurysms of femoral arteries are less common than diffuse dilatation of iliac and common femoral arteries. Blood flow through the latter tends to be brisk. Aneurysms may rupture, loosen emboli, or promote stenoses secondary to kinking at the junction of both intact and diseased arteries. Enlarging focal aneurysms of the femoral artery warrant operative removal and replacement of the segment. Physical examination may fail to disclose aneurysms of the superficial femoral artery. Their removal simultaneously with aneurysms of common femoral or popliteal arteries appears reasonable. Focal aneurysms of the profunda femoris artery have not been recognized.

Profunda femoris arteries are the principal conduits of blood into distal vessels in the frequent circumstances of pathologic processes in superficial femoral arteries. Stenoses at their origins may be focal or may extend into branches. Discrete stenoses commonly occur in branches. All these lesions are susceptible to repair which may preclude more extensive operations as well as restore comfort and nutrition to distal parts. Dissection discloses the parallel course of the profunda femoris artery immediately posterior and lateral to the superficial femoral artery. Experience convinces the surgeon of the ease and satisfactory consequences of reconstructive operations upon the profunda femoris artery, and angiography corroborates this optimism.

Atherosclerotic involvement of the bifurcation of the common femoral artery presents a spectrum of pathology which may be treated a number of ways. Improved practices will evolve as evaluation by angiography and measurement of blood flow illustrates shortcomings of prior and current surgical measures. Presumably the least technical difficulty is created by placing occluding clamps with broad blades on relatively soft parts of arteries. When incision into the common femoral artery is made for insertion of an aorta-femoral bypass graft, for the origin of a femoral-popliteal graft, or for local embolectomy or throm-bectomy, the surgeon selects the least sclerotic site. Deliberate incision avoids separation of layers. Local endarterectomy is *not* done. The arteriotomy site is held open by 5-0 traction sutures placed 4 to 6 mm from the cut edge.

The importance of the circular constricting effect of the plaque at the orifice of the profunda femoris artery has been appreciated, but it is probable that considerably more attention to the profunda femoris artery routinely will improve circulation to the extremity. Occlusion of the superficial femoral artery and angiographic or palpable evidence of plaque in the proximal millimeters of the profunda femoris artery necessitates an oblique incision extending from the distal common femoral artery into the profunda femoris artery. The effect is that of a wide lumen as the distal limit of the graft functionally becomes a composite graft. At times the atherosclerotic process extends into bifurcations of the pro-funda. Suboptimal care can cause thrombosis, which is to be avoided by assess-ment of angiograms or the tributaries themselves and by appropriate care. When the process is focal, temporary occlusion of arteries distal to the sclerotic segments permits separate incisions, endarterectomy, and reconstruction (Fig. 4-48). An alternative solution is also applicable to instances of diffuse atherosclerosis of tributaries. Red rubber catheters of appropriate caliber are introduced into tribu-taries to preclude back-bleeding, while endarterectomy is terminated smoothly within the larger vessel. A long narrow segment of the main trunk of the profunda femoris artery may be managed better by incision, superficial sculpturing (scrap-ing), and closure primarily, or with a venous patch graft, than by blind or open endarterectomy (Figs. 4-49 and 4-50).

Procedures little used to date may be considered for bypass graft into the profunda femoris artery, or for autograft of the excised common femoral artery. Endarterectomy of the common and profunda femoris artery cannot ignore the thrombogenic surface presented by the occluded orifice of the superficial femoral artery. It is easy to divide the latter a few centimeters from its origin and perform endarterectomy in continuity with the common femoral artery. The site of division of the superficial femoral artery may be determined by the length necessary for use as a bypass graft into the distal profunda femoris artery (Fig. 4-51). The prox-imal superficial femoral artery has been incised on its anterior aspect in continuity with the incision of the common femoral artery and folded proximally to effect a composite patch graft reconstruction. A segment of occluded superficial femoral artery may be excised, its obstruction removed, and this autograft used as a tubular connection between the common and profunda arteries in rare instances when the bifurcation is excised. In all instances this segment of artery is useful for arteri-otomy for termination or origination of bypass grafts.

Less than optimal caliber of the profunda femoris artery may be caused by clamping its sclerotic wall with the mistaken notion that dilatation or calibration with a catheter or instrument will restore the plaque intima that was deformed and disrupted by application of arterial clamps. It is better to be realistic in ack-nowledging the probability of clamps causing trauma and avoid their use by inserting catheters to preclude back-bleeding. The consequences of fracture of plaques must be assessed by angiogram or corrected by endarterectomy and/or patch graft.

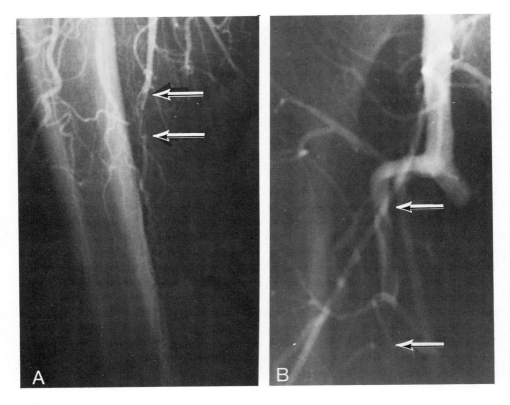

Figure 4-48. FOCAL LESION IN PROFUNDA FEMORIS ARTERY. (A, B) Interruptions of profunda femoris artery are to be removed by balloon catheter, if embolic or thrombotic, and by direct operative exposure, if atherosclerotic. Scrape endarterotomy or onlay patch graft may be used.

Previously only the common femoral artery was isolated and clamped to install the proximal limb of a femoral-distal bypass graft. It appears wiser to acknowledge the not inconsiderable possibility of failure of reconstruction of femoral arteries and prepare the profunda to maintain viability of the entire extremity. This will become increasingly popular as the contiguity of the superficial and profunda femoris arteries is appreciated. Rarely are these arteries farther apart than is apparent on angiography. Minimal medial retraction of the superficial femoral artery is required. The occasional venous branch traversing the course of the profunda may be spared or used for patch grafts. The caliber of the profunda femoris artery permits reconstructive procedures, and the measured quantities of blood it can conduct demands greater utilization of it in surgical reconstruction.

The most common artery selected for operative reconstruction has always been the superficial femoral artery. Evidence is cited that obstruction in it alone rarely causes symptoms. The onus for symptoms from reduced circulation to the leg must be placed upon coincident arterial stenoses proximal and distal to the

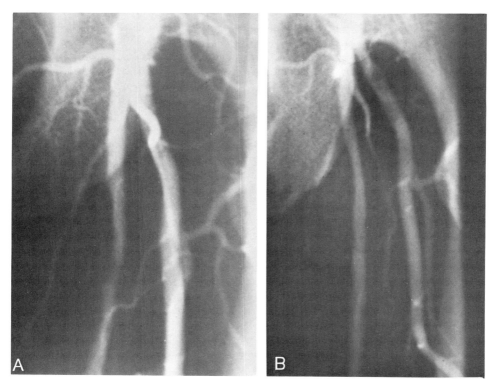

Figure 4-49. PARTIAL THICKNESS ENDARTERECTOMY. (A) Diffusely narrowed superficial femoral artery has focal near-total occlusion. (B) Postoperative angiogram following partial thickness endarterectomy, by technique seen in Figure 4-50.

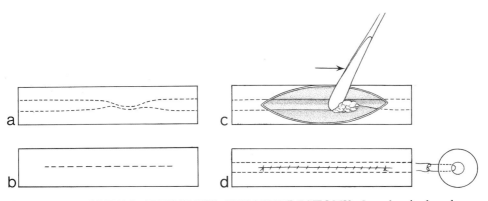

Figure 4-50. PARTIAL THICKNESS ENDARTERECTOMY. Intraluminal enlargement by surface abrasion may be useful when prophylaxis or salvage are virtually demanded in vessels too diseased for elective procedures with standard techniques. This reluctantly performed maneuver may achieve an end-result sought by rarely-practiced intraluminal dilatation (see Figure 4-49).

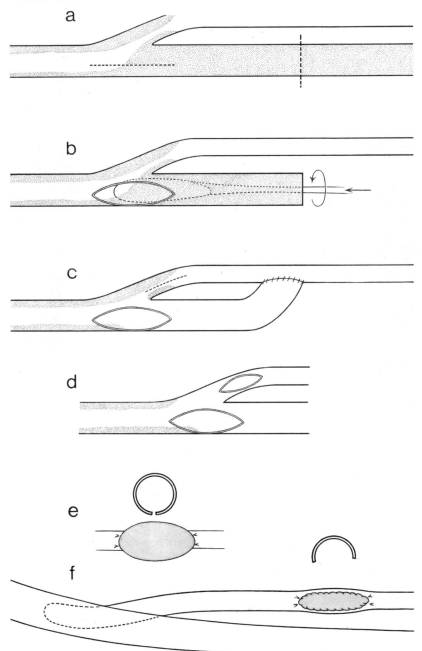

Figure 4-51. ENDARTERECTOMY, BYPASS, AND PATCH GRAFT. Endarterectomy of proximal portion of occluded superficial femoral artery may yield conduit with which to bypass stenotic segments of deep femoral artery (c). An incision opposite the orifice of deep femoral artery obviates imprecise technical results (a, b, c). This plus endarterectomy of tributary artery provides two useful channels (d). If vein or prosthetic material is used as patch graft, discarding some of the circumference of the graft and inclusion of liberal cuff of patch (f) precludes disproportion (e) and its attendant turbulent flow.

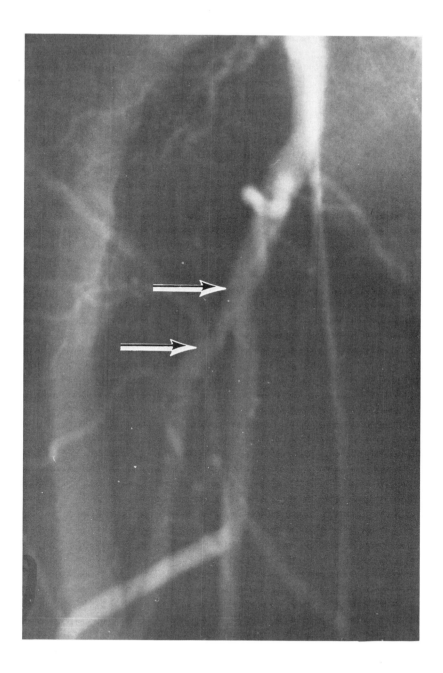

Figure 4-51 (cont.). Angiogram illustrates stenotic proximal portion of branch of profunda femoris artery (arrows), amenable to endarterectomy.

superficial femoral artery. Nonetheless, necrotic lesions, rest pain, and pronounced claudication have been benefited greatly and permanently by limited operations upon superficial femoral arteries. This soft tissue operation is well tolerated, involving minimal morbidity when successful. Many surgeons believe that bypass grafts which fail rarely obstruct the segment of lumen distal to sites of implantation of graft, while thrombosis in segments treated by endarterectomy extends proximally and distally and obstructs collateral arteries. Thus, segmental occlusions with large caliber in-flow and run-off vessels are indications for femoral artery restoration without concomitant iliac reconstruction. Iliac reconstruction alone is preferred when popliteal vessels above the knee joint appear unsuited to restoration of primary circulation (see discussion, p. 115).

EMBOLECTOMY FROM COMMON FEMORAL ARTERY.   The frequent lodging of embolus in the distal common femoral artery invites description of technical considerations. The caliber of the common femoral artery permits entrance of embolus, while narrower lumina of superficial and deep femoral arteries precludes exit. Prior to incision in the larger artery, a portion of superficial femoral artery is isolated and obstructed, to trap the embolus and to preclude passage distally of the fragments in toto. Isolation of the deep femoral artery is desirable, and experience with the technique accomplishes that maneuver easily. A portion of common femoral artery, approximately an inch proximal to the profunda, is isolated for control of flow through it, but the artery is *not* occluded until incision, embolectomy, and spontaneous flushing have taken place. Incision is made into the common femoral artery opposite the origin of the deep femoral artery. The embolus frequently extrudes itself if it is small, aided by force of arterial pressure and retraction of muscular arterial wall. When the embolus is long, and it or thrombus formation continues to obstruct the vessel proximally, the distal fragment is manipulated first. With broad forceps, this is drawn proximally into the arteriotomy incision to note whether distal arterial pressure via collateral circulation will aid its extrusion from superficial and deep branches. The longitudinal incision may be lengthened, extending the view of the operative field in either direction as necessary. If back-bleeding is brisk from major branches, it seems meddlesome to introduce a catheter for aspiration, irrigation, or manipulation. If back-bleeding from the deep femoral artery is not at the rate and volume anticipated, this artery is dissected to its bifurcation. When palpable thrombus is present, a balloon catheter should be introduced via the arteriotomy site and orifice and guided past the obstruction prior to inflation of the balloon and withdrawal of the catheter. The second branch may be explored similarly. If there is not ready access to the continuation distally of the deep femoral artery, there is justification for trial probing to achieve calibration and back-bleeding.

Thrombus proximal to the embolus is removed by introducing a balloon catheter a measured distance into the external iliac artery to be certain its tip is proximal to the embolus prior to inflation and withdrawal. If routine angiography was not done prior to operation, there are differences of opinion and practice concerning use of balloon catheters. The balloon catheter should not be inserted as high as the iliac bifurcation to preclude impacting the thrombus into the hypogastric artery. Certainly it should not be passed to the aortic bifurcation, to avoid dislodgement of obstructing material into arteries of the opposite side. When proximal flow is satisfactory, closure of the arteriotomy site and palpation for distal pulses is advocated rather than routine passage of balloon catheters. Closure without constriction is possible, as is enlargement with patch graft if the arterial wall became disrupted by coarse manipulation. If a distal pulse is not palpable despite preoperative angiographic evidence of arterial patency, 10 cc of 1 percent procaine and/or 30 mg of papaverine may be injected into the artery. (Of course, it is assumed that normal systemic arterial and central venous pressures exist at this time.)

Angiography at operation discloses sites and extent of patency and of obstruction, guiding placement of subsequent incisions. If there is obstruction, *principle requires exposure of the next bifurcation,* that is, the bifurcation of the popliteal artery below the knee. This is done by placing an incision in the medial aspect of the proximal leg and another in the popliteal artery opposite the anterior tibial artery. Surgical control of the popliteal artery precludes distal embolization, and permits embolectomy-thrombectomy of the superficial femoral artery by the technique of retrograde flush, retrieving embolus and thrombus through the reopened femoral arteriotomy site. This technique, when applicable and successful, can remove thrombotic obstruction from collateral vessels. The extended specimen may be a cast with many prongs representing sites of arterial branches. If the flush technique is unsuccessful but arterial caliber is favorable, mechanical thrombectomy with balloon catheter or other scraping dilating device can remove embolus (thrombus) and restore conditions conducive to flow.

Choosing to place the next distal arteriotomy site beyond the common femoral artery at the adductor canal has been the incorrect practice of many surgeons, based upon unfamiliarity with anatomy and fear of results of operation upon vessels of lesser caliber distal to the knee. Even if atheromatous involvement of the femoral artery at the adductor canal contributes to lodging of embolus there and/or propagation of thrombus in either direction, nonmanipulative evaluation of that site by angiography is preferable to surgical exploration of the distal thigh. At times angiography for complications of emboli discloses classic atherosclerotic obstruction in the superficial femoral artery, with patency beyond it. In these instances arterial reconstruction is required, and the incision in the medial aspect of the distal thigh is correct for performance of endarterectomy or bypass graft.

EMBOLECTOMY IN SUPERFICIAL AND DEEP FEMORAL ARTERIES.   Emboli obstructing orifices of superficial and deep femoral arteries interrupt the normal resting blood flow of 10 to 15 percent of cardiac output, which is sorely missed. There is intense pain in the foot and calf, less in the thigh, a magnification of disabling rest pain and claudication suffered by patients with chronic occlusion. Coldness, loss of discriminatory sensation, paresis, and blanching occur early and progress. Skin discoloration is apparent distal to mid-thigh, beginning as far distally as the supracondylar level in some patients. Knowing that limb survival without restoration of circulation is impossible, and that ischemic symptoms demand relief, operation is advisable at once, irrespective of duration of occlusion or severe systemic disease. Occasionally, extraordinary primitive psychosocial circumstances of patients permit gangrene and shock to advance so that amputation or death appear inevitable. Formerly, administration of heparin systemically and refrigeration of the extremity appeared to be better judgment than arterial exploration, fearing such patients could not survive vascular operation or amputation prior to resuscitation. Current concepts of monitoring central venous pressure and blood gas composition as indices of adequacy of blood volume and cardiac responses to treatment make immediate concurrent resuscitation and definitive treatment logical "routine" procedure.

Occlusion of only the superficial femoral artery can cause coldness but rarely severe rest pain if deep femoral artery pathways remain patent. Coldness, parasthesias, pallor with elevation, absent pulses, and prolonged venous filling time attest the abnormal circulation which comprises function but rarely threatens viability. Spasm complicates embolic occlusion, intensifying ischemic symptoms and signs. Thrombosis may occlude collateral circulation and propagate distally and proximally, converting the functional circumstances to those of occlusion of the common femoral artery (rare) or of the popliteal artery. Good judgment favors operative restoration of circulation, even though viability permits non-operative therapy. There is scant justification for failure to restore flow through major arteries.

Pain in upper thigh and buttocks which is intensified by activity is consistent with embolic occlusion of the deep femoral artery, although previously such symptoms were ascribed almost exclusively to obstruction of the hypogastric artery. This clinical impression needs confirmation angiographically. Operative removal of embolus from the profunda femoris artery can relieve serious symptoms and is warranted.

POPLITEAL ARTERIES

Localized classic aneurysms of popliteal arteries require operation when discovered or symptomatic. Not uncommonly, popliteal aneurysms are bilateral, and the natural history of the symptomatic aneurysm (e.g., swelling, pain, ischemia, rupture) seems to suggest the desirability of correcting the second side even though asymptomatic (Fig. 4-52). End-results of operation generally are so favorable, and complications of spontaneous rupture, embolization, or thrombosis so dreaded, that commonly surgeons suggest and patients accept treatment of the second aneurysm. Spontaneous thrombotic occlusion of popliteal aneurysms causing ischemic symptoms requires distal revascularization, not necessarily excision of the aneurysm. Occlusion of the aneurysm and threatened gangrene of the foot or leg requires operative exploration and angiography of arteries distal to the aneurysm to effect thrombectomy and/or reconstructive operation. Revascularization operations may be contraindicated for systemic reasons in the presence of advanced gangrene. Such procedures may be unnecessary when symptoms are mild, when necrosis is not a threat, and when activity of the patient lies within function of the extremity. Not infrequently, unexpected complications have jeopardized limbs sooner than imagined.

Atherosclerotic stenoses or occlusions of the popliteal artery merit operation when ischemic symptoms, signs, and disability are marked, and when caliber, wall, and patency of distal vessels offer technical feasibility and adequate run-off. Cellulitis, fissure, ulcer, and gangrene of the heel, toe, lateral malleolus, or site of the head of the fifth metatarsal compromise borderline circulation and foretell amputation, unless marked improvement in blood supply is achieved. Claudication and rest pain are cause for operation if the anatomy of distal vessels is so favorable that a successful outcome of operation is virtually assured. At the other extreme, vessels with minimal diameters of lumina and x-ray evidence of calcium in walls offer scant probability of long-term patency, and operation should *not* be attempted. The availability of saphenous vein for use as grafts may offer greater chance of prolonged patency than cloth prosthetic graft material (Fig. 4-53). Thus, borderline indications for operation incur higher risk if the graft material is not autogenous, and if synthetic material must cross the knee joint to be sutured to vessels with small caliber and porcelain-like walls. Decreased caliber and intimal fibrosis of saphenous veins occurs commonly in patients with diffuse severe sclerosis of femoral and popliteal arteries. Here is a place for judgment

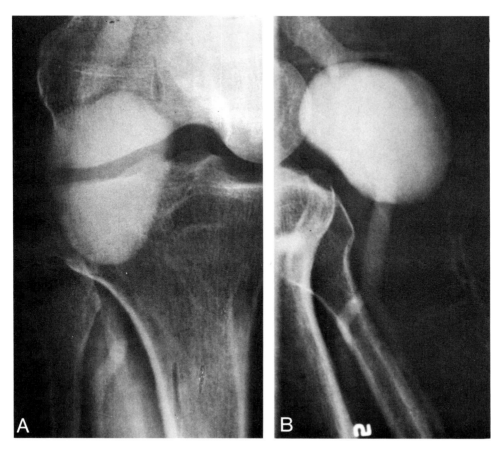

Figure 4-52. POPLITEAL ARTERY ANEURYSMS. (A, B) AP and lateral angiograms of one of paired popliteal artery aneurysms in a 74-year-old man.

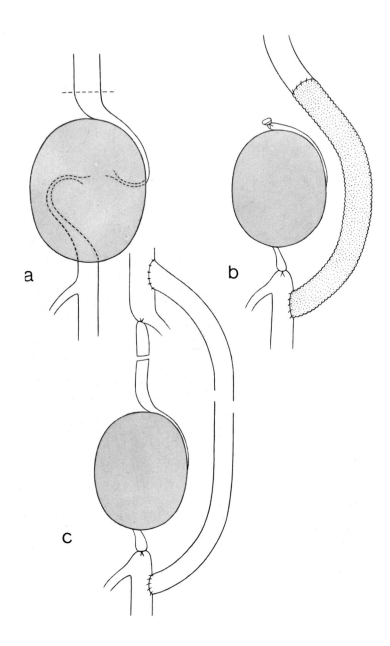

Figure 4-52 (cont.). Drawing depicts aspects of pathophysiology of aneurysm in a confined space—elongation as well as transverse enlargement of artery (a). Thrombus material in the lumen and extraluminal compression, rotation and distortion of afferent and efferent portions of artery diminish rate of flow. Bypass grafts, regional with prosthetic material on one side, and femoral-popliteal with autogenous vein on the other side, have given asymptomatic results for more than five years. High pressure communications with aneurysms were interrupted, as depicted (b, c).

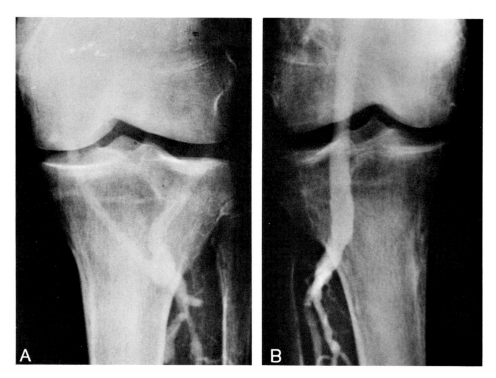

Figure 4-53. GRAFT INSERTIONS DISTAL TO KNEE. (A) Cloth bypass graft to popliteal artery below the knee joint line. (B) Vein bypass graft terminating in popliteal artery below knee. (The large caliber of popliteal artery is unusual, except in association with popliteal artery aneurysm). Each run-off vessel has high-grade stenoses, yet both grafts in same patient have functioned more than four years.

and preparedness. When vein distal to the knee does not enlarge to 4 mm or more by hydrostatic dilatation, the failure rate may be expected to exceed 75 percent. Autogenous cephalic vein or venous allografts may be used with high expectation of prolonged success. A less satisfactory alternative is early termination of such an exploratory operation, to minimize disservice to patients and to the reputation of arterial surgery. Patients' limbs may still bear them, or unavoidable amputations may be performed without delay.

Popliteal artery occlusion may occur at several sites, and the relation of the obstruction to the several levels of collateral vessels determines clinical outcome (Fig. 4-54). Superior and middle geniculate arteries arise 4 and 3 inches above the knee joint line, respectively, and communicate with inferior geniculate and tibioperoneal vessels (Fig. 4-55). Emboli which lodge at or above these collateral vessels produce severe ischemia of the leg. Ischemia is less severe and consistent with viability when emboli lodge between collateral vessels; least functional disability is incurred when an embolus lodges near the knee joint line. Atherosclerotic plaques may trap emboli which have passed natural barriers (i.e., bifurcations) proximally.

Figure 4-54 (left). POSTERIOR EXPOSURE OF POPLITEAL ARTERY. The femoral artery approaches the popliteal space from the medial aspect of the distal thigh. Anterior emergence of the anterior tibial artery, lateral to the tibia, obligates a lateral course of the distal popliteal artery. The flexion crease in the skin may be several centimeters distal to the joint line.

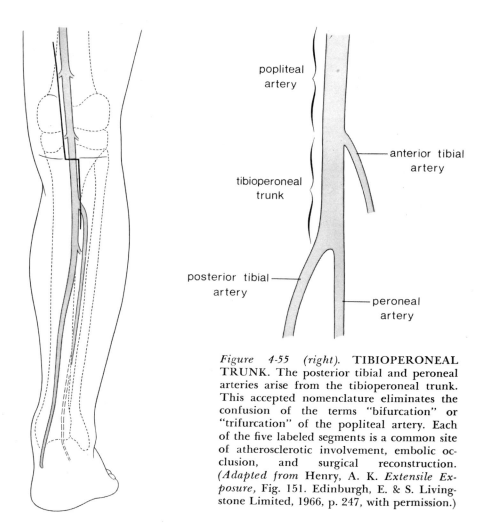

Figure 4-55 (right). TIBIOPERONEAL TRUNK. The posterior tibial and peroneal arteries arise from the tibioperoneal trunk. This accepted nomenclature eliminates the confusion of the terms "bifurcation" or "trifurcation" of the popliteal artery. Each of the five labeled segments is a common site of atherosclerotic involvement, embolic occlusion, and surgical reconstruction. *(Adapted from* Henry, A. K. *Extensile Exposure,* Fig. 151. Edinburgh, E. & S. Livingstone Limited, 1966, p. 247, with permission.)

Figure 4-56. (a) This drawing illustrates placement of incision at plane of posterior aspect of tibia, just behind the not-so-prominent posterior-medial surface of tibia. (b) The greater saphenous vein lies along the course of incision and is not to be injured. Its branches coursing anteriorly or posteriorly aid identification of its location. Fascia deep to it is incised. (c) Blunt dissection beneath incised fascia locates popliteal artery, vein, and nerve. A Cloward laminectomy retractor exposes the area. Sharp dissection isolates anterior and posterior tibial arteries and peroneal artery. Saphenous vein or prosthetic grafts are anastomed to popliteal artery proximal to anterior tibial artery, obligating entry virtually at right angles to host artery (d).

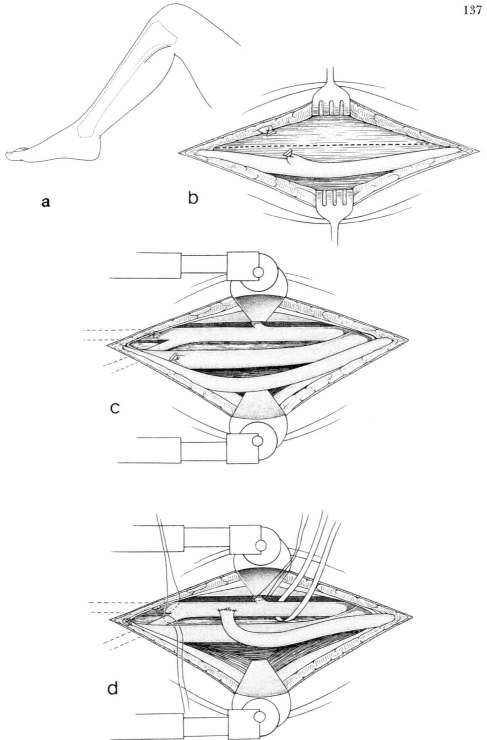

Figure 4-56. EXPOSURE OF VESSELS OF PROXIMAL LEG
(POPLITEAL TRIFURCATION)

Occlusion of popliteal artery distal to the knee joint, obstructing the anterior tibial artery and tibioperoneal trunk, produces severe ischemic disability and leads to a high incidence of limb loss. Discoloration and temperature change is obvious at mid-leg. Knee motion is intact, while ankle and toe motions are more severely restricted. Popliteal pulse may be present, even bounding. **Careful note must be taken of the most distal site of pulsation relative to the joint line,** lest the examiner fail to appreciate the probable actual level of arterial obstruction and the need for early restorative operation.

All popliteal artery emboli warrant serious consideration of removal by direct operative exposure of the bifurcation of the popliteal artery. There is every likelihood of successful restoration of normal circulation when the popliteal artery is the most distal site occluded by embolus. Gangrene and amputation are threatened when tibial arteries are occluded. The thrombogenic nature of intrinsic arterial disease and the sparseness of collateral circulation between geniculate arteries and tibioperoneal vessels contribute to the high rate of early thrombosis in arteries of the leg when the popliteal artery is obstructed with embolus which is not removed promptly.

The known high rate of loss of leg and foot in instances of acute occlusion of popliteal arteries effectively counterbalances relative contraindications of popliteal artery embolectomy. It is fortunate that popliteal and femoral artery exposures are easy and are well tolerated with local anesthesia. With the patient supine and the knee supported by sheets in a position of 30 degrees flexion, 0.5 percent xylocaine is injected into skin and fascia preparatory to a 3-inch curvilinear incision placed 1 cm posterior to the anteromedial edge of the tibia (Fig. 4-56). The most proximal portion of this incision is 1 inch distal to the joint line. Care is taken to avoid injury to the saphenous vein. It is helpful when a venous tributary is exposed, for it may be traced to the parent vein prior to possible inadvertent division. The fascia encompassing calf muscle is incised, and popliteal areolar tissue yields at once to the exploring index finger. The absence of pulsation does not hamper identification of the artery because of the constant course of the anterior tibial artery, proceeding anteriorly between both leg bones cephalad of the interosseous membrane. Frequently several venous branches cross medial to the tibioperoneal trunk, and these must be sought, ligated, and divided to achieve visibility of the posterior tibial and peroneal arteries. Prior to anteriotomy, 2-0 silk ligatures are passed loosely around the arteries. Heparin is given intravenously and repeated at intervals. Incision is made on the posteromedial aspect of the junction of the popliteal artery and tibioperoneal trunk, opposite the orifice of the anterior tibial artery, more than 90 degrees rotation from it (Figs. 4-57, 4-58). Each artery is released transiently to flush the embolus or thrombus. Apparently adequate flow from each encourages suturing of the arteriotomy to restore blood flow and to permit examination for restoration of pulses. Few surgeons can resist the impulse to insert Fogarty or newer-concept balloon catheters measured distances into posterior tibial, peroneal, anterior tibial, and popliteal arteries, in that order. But that may be wrong!

Failure to restore distal pulses warrants angiography. It is incorrect to invoke spasm as the mechanism interfering with pulsatile flow. Retrograde flush by passage of an irrigating catheter or by insertion of a needle into exposed

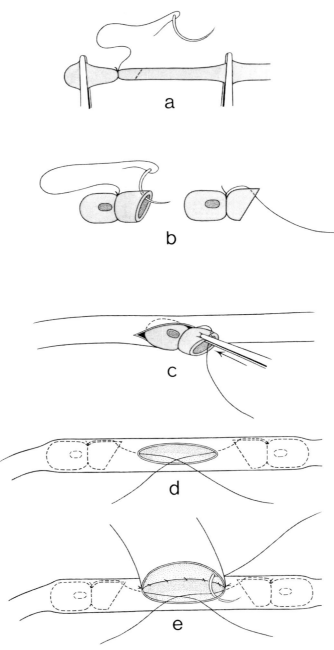

Figure 4-57. INTRALUMINAL OCCLUDING STENTS. A red rubber catheter of appropriate size (e.g., 8 Fr.) is stretched and tied with 2-0 silk, occluding its lumen (a). Site of knot determines location of long end of bevel which accepts suture to aid withdrawal of stent (b). Gentle transient occlusion of arterial segment with broad forceps permits arteriotomy and insertion of catheter tips (c). The catheter tips obviate application of clamps (and their trauma), dilate vessel (minimally), and expose inside of full circumference of arteriotomy site for careful and precise placement of each suture (d, e).

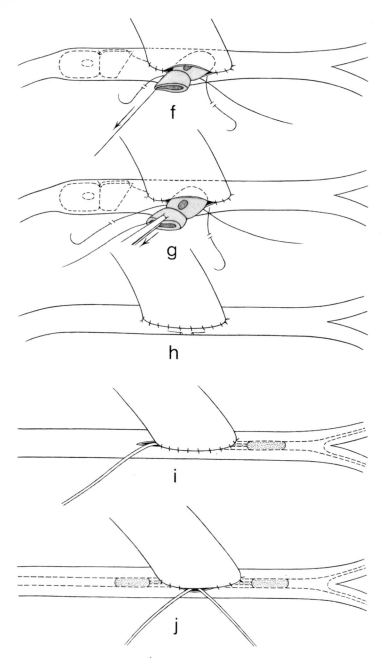

Figure 4-58. INTRALUMINAL OCCLUDING STENTS. When "plugs" are removed (f, g) there is excellent apposition of graft with host, minimizing bleeding as final two sutures are placed and tied.

Alternative procedures: In tiny arteries (e.g., coronary arteries) or in arteries with thick plaques and small lumina (e.g., salvage procedures in arteries distal to knee), size 8 Fr. catheters may be too large. Fogarty catheters may be inserted and balloons inflated. This is far more costly than rubber catheters, and presence in arteriotomy site is a bit of a nuisance (i, j). When only one direction from arteriotomy site is patent (i) catheter may lie in longer-than-necessary tract. The latter is closed after graft has been anastomosed and catheter withdrawn.

Figure 4-59. RETROGRADE FLUSH EMBOLECTOMY. Inability to advance Fogarty catheters to completely clear thrombi from anterior and posterior tibial arteries, coupled with ischemic, imperilled appearance of foot may lead surgeons to open small arteries distally to permit forceful retrograde irrigation. The perfusate distends arterial walls and the freed embolus-thrombus is extruded through a proximal arteriotomy incision (b).

The configuration of the Medicut® catheter permits its use as a dilator (a, c) to symmetrically enlarge the caliber of two ends of a small artery to aid precise approximation of edges and reconstruction of lumen (d).

But, perfection may be the enemy of good. Failure to clear lumen proximally precludes pressure and flow necessary to maintain patency distally (Fig. 4-60). Irrespective of condition or technique, operative angiography makes an all-important contribution toward achieving the desired result of assured restoration of flow through nonthrombogenic lumina.

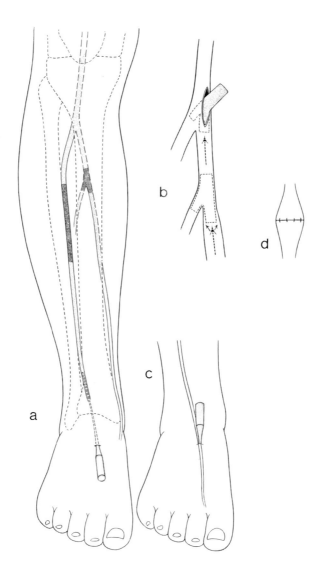

posterior tibial or dorsalis pedis arteries and instillation of warm saline may be preferred to "blind" antegrade introduction of catheters for aspiration or extraction of thrombus (Fig. 4-59). The mechanism by which retrograde flush may ease thrombus from bifurcations and tributaries is by fluid distention of arteries circumferentially away from thrombus, "floating" the thrombus cephalad. Opportunity to accomplish this almost certainly is lost once intra-arterial instrumentation has been unsuccessful in removing thrombotic material. If antegrade manipulation fails to remove all thrombus and embolus, side-effects are fragmentation and tamponade of thrombus material, or dissection and disruption of arterial wall.

Absent foot pulses but retained sensation, motion, and near-normal temperature and color of skin indicate that viability and function are likely to be retained. However, angiography in the operating room definitely is indicated to determine the site and extent of interference with circulation to permit inference of ease of operative restoration of circulation. The surgeon may be tired or discouraged, but the systemic condition of the patient both allows and demands that circulation be restored. Nonpulsatile flow from the proximal popliteal artery requires angiography, retrograde flush, or manipulation of balloon catheters. Retrograde flushing is accomplished by inserting in retrograde direction a catheter nearly the caliber of the popliteal artery, tightening a tape around it, and injecting warm saline in small spurts, awaiting injection of obstructing material via the open femoral arteriotomy site. If angiography prior to arteriotomy disclosed a short segment of popliteal occlusion, a balloon catheter may be introduced retrograde and made (by measurement) to pass the proximal site of obstruction. The balloon is inflated to intraluminal caliber and withdrawn. If angiography demonstarted occlusion of much of the length of the femoral artery, the balloon catheter may be introduced via the femoral arteriotomy site, passed to the popliteal arteriotomy, inflated, and withdrawn. In both instances, the collateral vessels must be spared the complication of impacting thrombus into them. The aim of both maneuvers is to remove the clot from the orifices of collateral vessels, as well as from the principal channel. Retrograde flush is likely to effect this more completely than catheter thrombectomy.

Complications result from failure to restore circulation. This is culpable when intrinsic circumstances favored restoration, but information that might have been helpful was not used (e.g., angiography) or oversight of some detail contributed to incomplete restoration or early rethrombosis.

TIBIAL AND PERONEAL ARTERIES

Anterior tibial, posterior tibial, and peroneal arteries with demonstrated continuity distally into the foot may be used to revascularize extremities. Vessel continuity may be direct or by collateral circulation. Frequently segments of large caliber but short length of each of the three leg arteries communicate and progressively carry blood to the foot. Optimal prospects of success exist when lumina of these distal vessels apparently are normal by angiogram. Exploratory operation is justified to determine suitability of distal arteries as recipient sites for grafts when angiographic portrayal encourages reconstruction. Such attempts to relieve

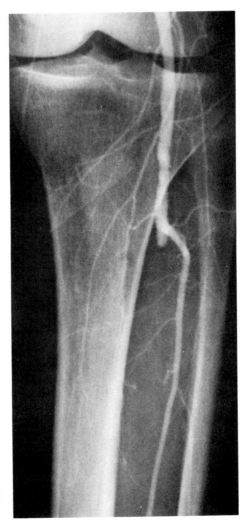

Figure 4-60. OCCLUSION OF TIBIOPER-
ONEAL TRUNK AND ITS BRANCHES.
Note irregularities of popliteal artery, which
have the appearance of trauma inflicted by
vascular clamps. Naturally occurring "ulcerating" lesions may look like this; thrombogenesis and arterioarterial emboli may be
consequences.

disabling symptoms and threatened tissue loss are warranted. Operation should
not be attempted when satisfactory angiograms disclose unfavorable circumstances; exploration in lieu of angiography is condemned.

Sudden interruption of circulation to the leg due to obstruction at the
bifurcation of the popliteal artery is more common than that due to lodging of
embolus in the tibioperoneal trunk or in just one of the three arteries of the leg.
However, instances of single vessel occlusion do occur (Fig. 4-60). When the
anterior tibial artery is occluded, the anterior compartment of dorsiflexing muscles
of the ankle and toes may manifest rest pain and weakness. Sensory effects are
minimal and changes in temperature and color do not often occur, but swelling
and tenderness may be obvious over the anterior compartment. The dorsalis pedis
pulse is diminished or is absent. Ischemic effects (neuropathy, swelling) have

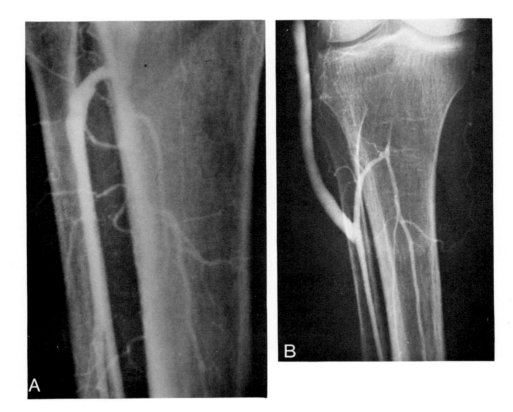

Figure 4-61. BYPASS GRAFTS TO ANTERIOR TIBIAL ARTERY. (A) Arteriotomy without endarterectomy: onlay vein patch graft reconstruction. (B) Anterior tibial insertion of reversed saphenous vein bypass graft. Vein lies in subcutaneous tunnel over anterolateral aspect of thigh.

been feared to the extent that incision of fascia has been advocated, hoping to relieve pressure and minimize compressive effects of edema. Three alternatives appear preferable: (1) angiography to define the site and extent of arterial occlusion to permit a plan of revascularization; (2) avoidance of procedures that contribute further to ischemic compression of anterior compartment (e.g., retrograde flushing); and (3) rest to minimize nutritional requirement with elevation to promote drainage and to minimize the ill-effects of edema. Operation without angiogram is not justified. Advanced atherosclerotic process of the orifice, proximal, and entire course of the anterior tibial artery have been observed, and such patients are likely to benefit little or none from optimistic but ill-fated operation along a thrombosed-sclerosed vessel. If the dorsalis pedis artery is operated upon, its location immediately lateral to the extensor hallucis longus precludes a long incision. Introduction of a plastic-sheathed thin needle offers the likelihood of retaining patency past that point after withdrawal of needle, while the use of incision and sutures predilects thrombosis (Fig. 4-61).

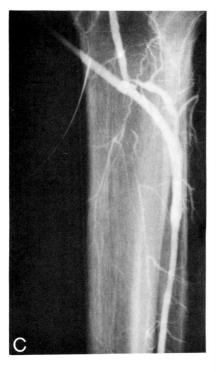
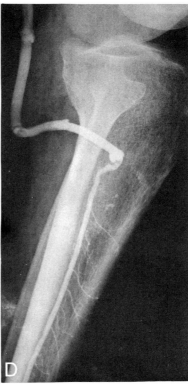

Figure 4-61 (cont.).   (C) Anterior tibial insertion of reversed vein graft. The vein coursed along its subcutaneous bed, across the medial approach to popliteal space, and into anterior compartment. Cephalad portion of interosseous membrane had been divided. (D) Saphenous vein bypass graft inserted into anterior tibial artery. This graft is considered too long. Anterior tibial artery exposure and reconstruction are easier at the junction of middle and upper thirds of leg. Each angiogram displays greater caliber of anterior tibial arteries, and absence of signs of trauma from clamps (intraluminal stents had been used).

Retrograde flushing via the dorsalis pedis artery into an unremediable artery may introduce and extravasate fluid with compressive effects upon collateral circulation. Such an artery may also be disrupted if intravascular instrumentation is used.

The anterior tibial artery is exposed high in the leg through a longitudinal incision placed midway between tibia and fibula (Fig. 4-62). Multiple small veins closely adherent to the artery may be mobilzed bloodlessly. Reconstruction of arteriotomy sites is aided by using a binocular magnifying loupe and 5-0 suture material. The wound is drained.

The posterior tibial artery is operated upon most commonly for embolic and thrombotic processes (Fig. 4-63). This artery is the straight-line continuation of the femoropopliteal system, and its size and accessibility behind the posterior

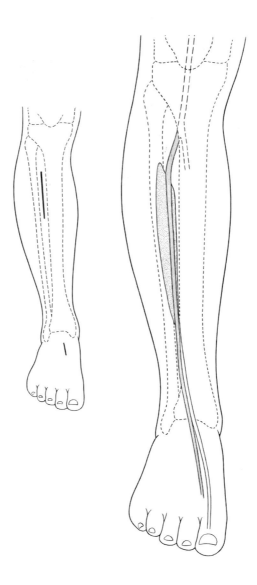

Figure 4-62. COURSE OF ANTERIOR TIBIAL ARTERY AND SITES OF OPER-ATIVE INCISIONS. Exposure of distal portion of proximal third of anterior tibial artery is accomplished through a longitudinal incision midway between tibia and fibula. This incision facilitates insertion of a bypass graft. Transverse incision near flexion crease of ankle or longitudinal on dorsum of foot locates artery lateral to tendon extensor hallucis longus.

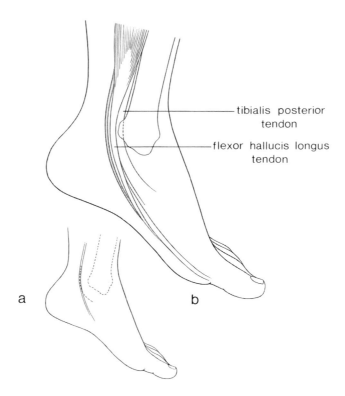

tibialis posterior
tendon

flexor hallucis longus
tendon

a   b

Figure 4-63. ARTERIOTOMY OF POSTERIOR TIBIAL ARTERY AT ANKLE. A
curvilinear incision on a 1.5 cm radius from posteroinferior aspect of medial malleolus
will permit ready exposure of artery for grafting or intraluminal manipulation.

malleolus encourages more optimism for patency after graft implantation than
for manipulation of thrombectomy. Estimates of failure to achieve patency are
imprecise, but such figures may be higher when operation is attempted only
after ill-effects have been produced by probing from above or below.

The peroneal artery recently has been advocated for operative exposure
and attempts at revascularization. Embolic occlusion of the bifurcation of the
tibioperoneal trunk may be relieved by passage of a balloon catheter into each
branch artery. If attempts to remove an embolus at that location are made by
passing a balloon catheter from the femoral or popliteal artery, success is rarer
(Fig. 4-64). Balloon catheter techniques directly dislodge the embolus mechanically
but may separate the embolus from the attached thrombus, or break the embolus
and thrombus into fragments. Incomplete removal can leave obstructing material,
and catheter manipulation can even tamp it into vessels (peroneal, tibial, or
collateral channels). Bypass grafts from the popliteal artery to the peroneal or
posterior tibial artery have relieved ischemia, salvaged extremities, or permitted
more distal amputation.

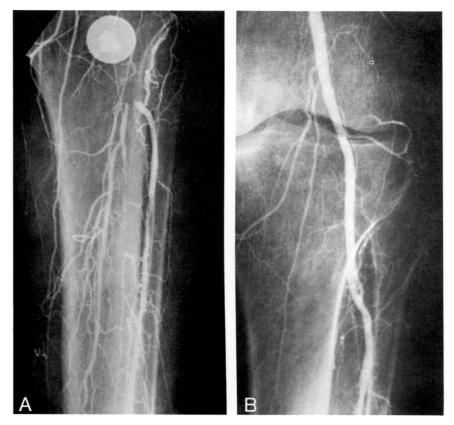

Figure 4-64. INCORRECT USE OF BALLOON CATHETER. (A) Thromboembolic occlusion of popliteal artery. Anterior tibial and tibioperoneal trunk and its tributaries are filled via collateral pathways. (B) Excellent restoration of popliteal artery caliber, but postembolectomy occlusion of tibioperoneal trunk and its branches. *Incorrect concepts* of sites of incisions in skin and arteries and *incorrect use* of Fogarty catheter caused this unsatisfactory result.

BYPASS GRAFTS TO POSTERIOR TIBIAL ARTERY AT ANKLE.   Bypass grafts from the common femoral to posterior tibial artery at the medial malleolus have achieved the status of standard procedures. The increasing experiences reported in the literature and our own limited but highly rewarding results of long-length bypass grafts encourages surgical reconstruction of vessels previously considered too small for routine successful technical management. Candidates for this procedure are patients with rest pain or ischemic skin lesions whose angiograms demonstrate unsuitable vessels for reconstruction at femoral, popliteal, and proximal tibial and peroneal levels. Patients previously denied operative reconstruction now may be reconsidered. Patients with embolic or thrombotic occlusions (in original or reconstructed segments) whose circulation is not successfully restored by the usual operative procedures at proximal sites may benefit from femoral-malleolar bypass reconstruction.

The following case history illustrates stages in thinking and progress in vascular surgery:

In 1964 in a metropolitan hospital, a 46-year-old diabetic male had bilateral operative exploration of femoral-popliteal arteries in the distal thighs, with division of adductor rings and of occluded arteries without relief of claudication. One year later in a university hospital, serial angiography disclosed occlusions of popliteal arteries, tibioperoneal trunks, and tibial and peroneal arteries in proximal portions of the legs, and the condition was considered unremediable. In 1968, claudication became more severe and rest pain began in one limb, and the patient noted absence of femoral artery pulse on that side. Angiogram was repeated with two objectives: demonstration of remediable sites of occlusion of iliac and proximal femoral arteries, and demonstration of arteries of the distal leg and foot. Optimal visualization of the latter may have been aided by hyperemia following release of cuff occlusion of the arteries of the thigh and by intra-arterial injection of 30 mg of papaverine 30 seconds prior to injection of 30 cc of 50 percent sodium diatrozoite (hypaque). Films were exposed at 2-second intervals for 30 seconds.

Angiographic findings were confirmed by operative exploration and postoperative angiogram. The posterior tibial artery was less than 2 mm in diameter behind the malleolus and was occluded 4 cm distally. Proximally there was patency to the lower third of the leg, with abundant communicaton with the distal anterior tibial artery. Together these vessels appeared to provide low-resistance large flow run-off, confirmed by continued long-term pulsatile function of autogenous saphenous vein bypass graft. Patency may have been encouraged by the large caliber of the vein, use of 7-0 silk and operating magnifying loupes, and intravenous infusion of low molecular weight dextran during and after operation.

COMPLICATIONS

Complications of vascular surgery may be systemic, regional, or local and commonly are related to both the disease process (atherosclerosis) and to suboptimal management of physiology or technique during or after operation.

Cerebral dysfunction may attend generalized hypoxia or hypercarbia, systemic hypotension of myocardial origin or blood loss, transient occlusion or permanent thrombosis of extracranial vessels, or hypertension induced by vasoactive agents or proximal cross-clamping of aorta.

Myocardial ischemia may be superimposed upon the substrate of significant stenoses of coronary arteries. Systemic hypotension, ventricular hypertension, and abnormal composition of blood (e.g., cold, acidotic, and hyperkalemic transfusion) may aggravate ischemia and intensify its consequences. Rapid release of clamps creating a large-capacity low-resistance reservoir, can interfere mechanically with myocardial contraction or cause abnormal rhythm.

Liver, kidneys, and intestines are organs with high metabolic rates and are vulnerable even to brief periods of hypoxia. Neural elements in extremities have time limts of tolerance to ischemia.

Extensive disease processes in small vessels impose limitations upon successful manipulation and repair. Deviant coagulation mechanisms (excess platelet adhesiveness) may increase the incidence of thrombosis even in larger vessels. Anticoagulaton may induce bleeding with dual abnormal effects of systemic hypotension or local compression interfering with flow. Embolic obstruction to flow is avoidable with proper sequence of operative manipulation.

Inadequate or inappropriate procedures may begin with diagnostic errors (minimized by appropriate suspicion, confirmed by angiography) and are affected by training, experience, and record of results of the surgeon. The local and regional pathology, as found and as created by surgical procedures, determines outcome. Embolectomy may be indicated but may not restore circulation if distal control of the vessel did not precede local manipulation, or if thrombosis was more extensive than appreciated. Ill-conceived "routine" maneuvers may be avoided by angiographic survey prior to unneeded manipulation.

Uncontrolled hemorrhage rarely occurs during operations by experienced vascular surgeons. Bleeding from preoperative rupture of aneurysms can be controlled, the outcome depending in part upon the mental and tactical preparedness of the surgeon and the hospital team. Hemorrhage secondary to disrupted infected sites of surgical closure or anastomosis are more difficult to control because arteries near infection become friable and may rupture during dissection to isolate and occlude them.

Mechanical disruption of vessels at sites of application of clamps or of anastomoses is rare unless bloodstream infection exists.

Wound hematoma is uncommon. Evacuation by reoperation is preferable to aspiration or manipulation, and prompt benign healing may be anticipated.

Thrombosis is related to vascular bed, surgical technique, and systemic hemodynamics. The majority of arteries operated upon probably offer the possibility of long-term patency. Thromboses in these vessels may be due to systemic hypovolemia and hypotension, but most often result from avoidable technical errors. Errors of judgment are considered technical, for their frequency can be minimized by objective evaluation of results (e.g., measurements of blood flow and operative angiography). Good case selection, technique, and physiologic maintenance of volume, flow, and pressure has virtually eliminated thrombosis early after arterial reconstruction.

Anticoagulant therapy has caused hemorrhage at all imaginable sites, with a frequency related inversely to attention given to details of dose and response. The benefits of effective anticoagulation when indicated are believed to outweigh the statistical incidence of complications. Most patients who develop hemorrhagic complications of anticoagulation therapy subsequently are manageable, and do receive anitcoagulants without complication. So many patients must be treated with anticoagulant drugs that physicians have no alternative to alert management.

Poor wound healing has been observed from extensive dissection of skin flaps and from trauma and desiccation of wound edges.

The highest incidence of infection in blood vessels is in relation to wound sepsis attending reconstructive surgical procedures. There is nothing unique about arterial operations predisposing to wound infection. However, incidence of wound infections increases in patients hospitalized longer than 14 days when hospital colonies of staphylococcus populate the environment and the person.

Infection in a wound through which arterial reconstruction was performed threatens hemorrhage, interruption of continuity of artery, loss of function and viability of the part, and death of the person. Blood-borne infections can localize in blood vessel walls and weaken them (mycotic aneurysm), threatening early or delayed rupture. Successful avoidance of disruption of infected artery may require many weeks of hospitalization for infusion of expensive antibiotics. The grounds for treatment may be empiric or well founded, and the decision not to treat unproved bacteremia or arteritis may cost organ, limb, or life. Infection may travel along the course of a prosthesis and involve multiple arteriotomy sites, threatening disruption concurrently at several locations, each with the grave implications of hemorrhage and shock, or at best ischemia distal to the site of arterial disruption.

Patients with congenital and acquired heart diseases are prone to blood stream infection, yet only rarely do such patients develop infection in a major blood vessel.

Breaks in surgical technique may occur in the operating room during preparation of skin and placement of drapes, gowns, and instruments, and by airborne contamination from nasopharyngeal bacteria of operating personnel. There are direct relationships between incidence of wound infection and deficiencies in patterns of air flow or in the filter system of the air-conditioning unit of an operating suite, the amount of talking by personnel, and the duration of the operation. Factors responsible for wound infection can affect the blood vessel or may cause wound infection only, sparing the blood vessel and its site of reconstruction. Hematoma or thrombosis which necessitate reoperation introduce a risk of contamination and infection. Endogenous infections (e.g., of the respiratory and urinary tracts) are considered important sources of bacteria responsible for wound infections. Distressing conditions for surgeons and potential threats to patients are incipient infections in arterial walls that do not become apparent while the operative wound heals. This complication may be overlooked until the patient has been discharged from the hospital. Fever, pain, expanding hematoma, external bleeding, or simply a draining sinus may occur. Hospitalization and intensive, prolonged antibiotic therapy are the least treatment; removal of graft and replacement via a circuitous route may become necessary.

RESULTS

In the literature the results of surgical operations are reported with honest intent but perhaps not without bias. This book presents the perspectives induced by our experiences. The follow-up results of operations in 110 patients performed consecutively *four to six years ago* upon arteries at various sites in the body are reviewed here.

CAROTID AND VERTEBRAL ARTERIES

Thirty-three patients had operations upon carotid and vertebral arteries to relieve symptoms and signs of cerebrovascular insufficiency; 20 patients had bilateral operations. Seven patients had operations upon nine vertebral arteries, each performed concurrently with carotid artery operation during the same anesthesia. Three patients had operations upon single vertebral arteries only.

Benefits of operation.   In 20 patients in whom the symptoms preceding operation were transient ischemic episodes of neurologic deficit, 15 were relieved completely, while three have complaints similar to those before operation. Twent-two patients (67 percent) had no complications during or after 39 operations.

Deaths.   Five patients died and six patients developed neurologic dysfunction while in the hospital. Two patients, aged 79 and 80, had bilateral occlusions of internal carotid arteries and bilateral high-grade stenoses of vertebral arteries. Each had recovered from coma and could walk with assistance prior to operation. In both these elderly patients, extensive atherosclerosis of subclavian arteries led to local technical complications and prolonged operations with thoracotomy by bypass grafts from aortas, and both patients died within one week. Two patients did not waken from general anesthesia following their second operations and each died in three days. Both had enjoyed uneventful courses following endarterectomy upon contralateral carotid arteries. Autopsy in one showed occlusion of the contralateral internal carotid artery where endarterectomy had been performed one week previously. Autopsy in the second patient failed to disclose cause of death. A 57-year-old man developed myocardial infarction and cardiac arrest during right brachial angiography the ninth day after operation upon the second side. Angiogram and autopsy disclosed patency of all reconstructed arteries.

Complications.   A 60-year-old woman wakened from general anesthesia for operation upon a second carotid artery with no greater neurologic deficit than existed prior to operation but become hypotensive and developed paralysis and coma in the recovery room four hours later. Hypotension (70 mm Hg systolic) had existed untreated until stroke occurred. The patient survived, but unsteadiness of gait is disabling; four years later she still requires assistance to walk.

A 54-year-old woman developed basilar artery insufficiency and grave disability nine days after the second operation upon carotid and vertebral arteries. Stenosis of one carotid and one vertebral artery had been relieved at each previous operation. Tendency toward hypotension had been combatted with plasmanate and neosynephrin infusions for these nine days. Three years later, the patient has aphasia and requires assistance to walk.

Two patients did not recover consciousness immediately, and these major neurologic deficits required prolonged rehabilitation. Two other patients were well for one week or longer after operation upon carotid arteries, when new symptoms appeared in vertebral-basilar distribution.

Three late deaths.   A 46-year-old woman entered the recovery room after waking from general anesthesia without neurologic dysfunction. Three hours later cardiac arrest developed under circumstances simlar to those recorded above. Hemiparesis, aphasia, and obtundation were permanent, and the patient died of pneumonia seven months later.

A 54-year-old woman entered the hospital five weeks after second carotid artery operation with infected disrupted arteriotomy site. The opposite internal carotid artery could not be opened at prior operation. Hypotension accompanying blood loss and acute and permanent ligation of this only remaining carotid artery were followed by coma and death four days later.

Contraindcations and cautions. The results of all operations for carotid and vertebral artery occlusions performed over a seven-year period were reviewed recently. The cases cited above are part of that review. Higher incidences of death and grave complications were related to advanced age, serious associated diseases (e.g., diabetes mellitus, diastolic hypertension, myocardial infarction), extensiveness of atherosclerotic involvement of extracranial and intracranial arteries, and postoperatively to the prevalence of hypotension. Accordingly, the two octogenarians (see above) might have been considered inoperable. It may be desirable to precede a second operation with angiographic assessment of the first artery treated by operation. Hypotension must be prevented by fixing arbitrary limits below which pressor drugs and volume expansion are mandatory features of postoperative treatment.

RENAL ARTERY STENOSES

Eight patients had arterial reconstructive operations for renal artery stenoses. Two women, ages 31 and 38, had unilateral fibromuscular hyperplasia resected and reconstructed by vein grafts. One woman and five men, ages 54 to 77, had atherosclerosis as the cause of the stenoses, and bilateral renal endarterectomy was performed in these six patients. All patients are alive at intervals to four years. Hypotension was cured in none, was lower in both young women, and did not progress in any. Blood urea nitrogen is not further elevated nor above 19 mg% in any.

Renin levels were determined in blood from both renal veins and in peripheral blood in five patients. Renal vein renin was minimally and moderately elevated in two young women with fibromuscular hyperplasia, and was low to minimally elevated in all patients with atherosclerosis as the cause of renal artery stenosis. It was not markedly elevated in any of these patients but it was ten to twenty times normal in two patents with acute renal artery occlusion and infarction of kidney requiring nephrectomy.

AORTA-ILIAC OCCLUSION

Twenty-one patients were operated upon and all left the hospital improved. In one patient there was disruption of infected suture line of aorta-iliac endarterectomy on the seventeenth postoperative day treated by resection and bifurcation graft. Staphcidal antibiotics had to be discontinued because of allergic reactions, and at home, eight weeks after the second operation, there was erosion between proximal suture line and duodenum, resulting in death. A late complication occurred at 14 months in a second patient when an infected site of anasto-mosis of one limb of a bifurcation graft disrupted at its point of insertion into the common femoral artery (Fig. 4-65). This was treated successfully by local ligation and excision of femoral artery bifurcation, and by iliac-popliteal bypass graft through the obturator foramen. Thirteen months after the second operation, thrombosis occurred in that long graft, due to three vessel occlusive disease below the knee demonstrated angiographically and in the amputation specimen. A late complication in a third patient was hepatitis from which the patient recovered.

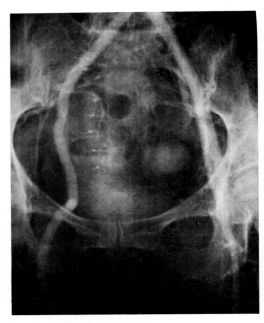 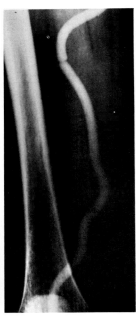

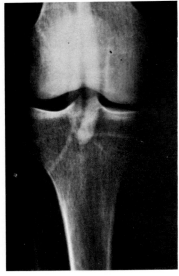

Figure 4-65. BYPASS OF INFECTED SITE THROUGH OBTURATOR FORAMEN. After 14 months of intermittent drainage from wound over right femoral triangle, disruption and hemorrhage occurred from the site of anastomosis between aorta-femoral graft and common femoral artery. Excision of infected site and ligation of arteries preceded anastomosis of tubular graft with limb of bifurcation graft and with tibioperoneal trunk.

The functional results of the group with occlusive lesions in both aorta-iliac and superficial femoral arteries is of great interest. Improvement followed the relief of proximal lesions in all instances, and has been so satisfactory that the wisdom of simultaneous operation distal to femoral arteries is questioned. Endarterectomy of the profunda femoris artery at its origin and at sites as far as three inches beyond the origin has been required commonly to affect these excellent functional results.

ABDOMINAL AORTIC ANEURYSMS

Abdominal aortic aneurysms were resected in 13 men and two women, ages 59 to 77. There were no instances of renal failure, myocardial infarction, congestive heart failure, or stroke complicating aneurysmectomy. Subsequently, additional operations were required in two patients with arterial embolic complications—popliteal artery in one and popliteal and mesenteric arteries in the second, the latter treated by resection of gangrenous bowel. These two patients died. Pulmonary embolism was suspected in one of these patients and was the proved cause of death in the other. Myocardial infarctions long after leaving the hospital and returning to work occurred in two patients who died within one year of aortic surgery.

FEMORAL-POPLITEAL GRAFTS

Cloth grafts, saphenous vein grafts, and in-situ saphenous vein grafts have maintained similar high patency rates for prolonged periods averaging two years. Failure to maintain patency in all groups appeared related to the severity of disease in distal arteries.

Twenty patients had bypass grafts between the common femoral artery and the popliteal artery proximal to the knee joint. Six of eight cloth grafts, all nine saphenous vein autografts, and two of three in-situ saphenous vein grafts maintained patency at 24 months.

In 13 patients, the distal site of insertion of femoral popliteal bypass grafts was below the knee. No thrombosis occurred in two saphenous autografts and in five in-situ saphenous vein grafts. Cloth grafts thrombosed at 6, 14, 28, and 38 months. One cloth and vein end-to-end graft thrombosed the day of operation.

POPLITEAL ARTERY

Popliteal aneurysmectomy and replacement with cloth or vein graft was uniformly successful in six patients. Popliteal endarterectomy with primary closure resulted in thrombosis in four months. The limb was salvaged by femoral-popliteal below-knee bypass graft with arteriovenous fistula (Fig. 4-66). Patency and distal palpable pulses continued 38 months, and a viable extremity without rest pain persists at four and one-half years. Five instances of popliteal endarterectomy with saphenous roof patches resulted in four long-term patencies and one occlusion at ten months. The occlusion occurred in a 30-year-old woman who simultaneously developed occlusion in the opposite popliteal artery despite its near-normal appearance at angiogram ten months earlier. Systemic disease manifested by microangiitis subsequently was proved in this patient.

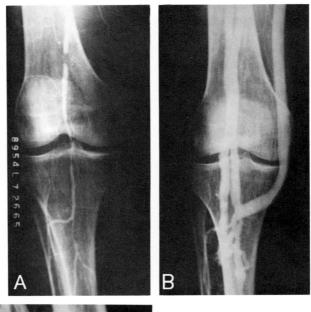

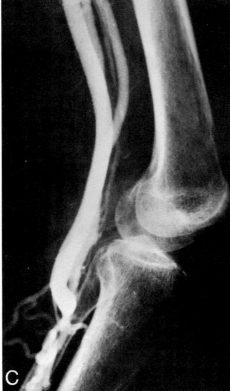

Figure 4-66. ARTERIOVENOUS FISTU-LA DISTAL TO GRAFT. (A) Occlusion of popliteal artery above knee and highgrade stenoses at and distal to joint line. Reconstruction by endarterectomy and vein patch graft rethrombosed in two months. Infected fissure of heel led to next operation. (B) Femoralpopliteal below-knee cloth bypass graft plus arteriovenous fistula created between tibioperoneal vessels. This remained patent 38 months. (C) Lateral view of B.

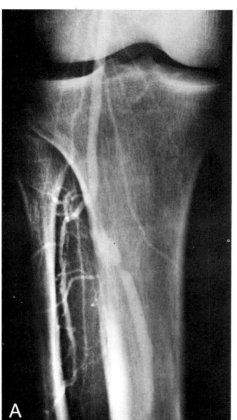

Figure 4-67. COMPRESSION OF VEIN GRAFTS BY ORGANIZING HEMA-TOMA. (A) Three weeks after femoral-posterior tibial bypass graft and (B) after femoral-peroneal graft. Lumen size and blood flow restored by explorations without incisions into grafts. Subsequently, in similar operations on other patients below-knee sites have been drained with sump-drainage for periods to 24 hours. (C) Demonstration of advanced atheromatous stenoses and occlusions present before reconstruction shown in B.

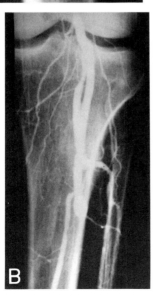

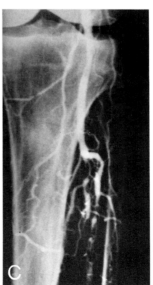

ANTERIOR TIBIAL ARTERY

Limited experiences with bypass grafts from femoral artery to anterior tibial artery were unfavorable, until technique became satisfactory. Limitations in technique were considered more important than length or caliber of graft. Doubtless poor selection and inadequate run-off into diseased distal vessels has contributed to early thromboses. Endarterectomy and patch graft reconstruction of the anterior tibial artery alone was successful in one instance (see Fig. 4-61, p. 144). Two patients with reconstructions that involved the tibioperoneal bifurcations and anterior tibial arteries developed thromboses, but patency into distal arteries was reestablished by saphenous vein bypass grafts.

PERONEAL ARTERY

Three instances of saphenous vein autografts between popliteal and peroneal arteries have maintained patency up to three years. The directness of the course of the graft and the conventional onlay end-to-side technique have been considered as important as the short length of the graft in contributing to maintained patency (Fig. 4-67).

RESULTS OF OTHERS' EXPERIENCES

CAROTID ARTERIES

Thompson[112] records 2.7 percent mortality in 748 operations upon 592 patients. MacDowell and his co-workers[6] reported 2 percent deaths and 2 percent new neurologic deficits in a recent series of 200 operations for carotid artery stenoses and occlusions in patients up to 80 years old. Rainer and his associates,[8] using cervical block anesthesia and electroencephalographic monitoring, found that 75 of 88 patients operated upon for cerebrovascular insufficiency due to atheromatous lesions in carotid arteries tolerated arterial occlusion. Ten of the remaining 13 were given physiologic adjuncts, and then tolerated operation without deterioration of EEG or new neurologic symptoms. DeBakey's report studying the relation between P_{ACO_2} and P_{AO_2} with general anesthesia and internal shunts in 45 patients cited one instance of postoperative stroke, caused by thrombosis postoperatively, relieved by reoperation.[10] DeBakey's series of 1,600 patients recorded 5 percent operative mortality and 6 percent morbidity, with relief of symptoms in 65 percent and improvement in an additional 20 percent.[3] Blaisdell and co-workers[106] noted that occluded internal carotid arteries may be opened in as many as 40 percent of cases, with maintained patency demonstrated angiographically in one-fifth.

CORONARY ARTERIES

Bypass grafts. Nearly uniform success has been achieved in a small series of patients in whom ends of internal mammary arteries were precisely anastomosed to arteriotomy sites in distal anterior descending coronary arteries. Blood flow measurements documented early and sustained increases in flow. Vein grafts between ascending oarta and coronary arteries are larger in caliber, carry more blood and may be expected to maintain patency in a high percentage of cases.

Endarterectomy. Earliest reports of May and Bailey[23] and of Longmire[27] cited higher operative mortality in reconstructive surgery of coronary arteries than the 25 percent recently reported by Effler.[24] A recent survey disclosed 10 percent mortality and 76 percent relief of symptoms following direct surgery on the coronary arteries of 278 patients. Long-term results of gas endarterectomy, advocated for the right coronary artery, are not yet available.

Myocardial implant of internal mammary artery. Angiography demonstrated functional arterial implants in 85 percent of instances at one year if stenoses greater than 90 percent existed in coronary arteries to areas of myocardium where internal mammary arteries had been implanted. The American College of Chest Physicians reported a survey of 120 surgeons who disclosed their results of myocardial revascularization.[22] There was an operative mortality of 6 percent of 2,255 patients when one internal mammary artery was implanted, 7.5 percent of 987 patients after bilateral implantation; 78 percent of the former and 63 percent of the latter groups obtained relief. Angiographic evidence of patency of implanted arteries and communication with regional coronary arteries was not reported.

ABDOMINAL VISCERAL ARTERIES

Morris and his colleagues[36] reported no mortality in 31 patients treated by operation for relief of visceral artery ischemia, noting all were better, and 90 percent were cured. Twenty-five of these patients had severe involvement of two of the three major arteries, and the celiac axis invariably was stenotic or occluded. Drapanas and Bron[35] observed 17 patients with stenosis or occlusion of celiac axis only. None of five patients operated upon was relieved of symptoms. Rob[37] reported higher patency rates from excision with graft replacement (81 percent) than with endarterectomy (50 percent). Szilagyi[38] reported only one survivor among 20 patients operated upon for acute occlusion of superior mesenteric artery. It appears necessary to relate this to delay in diagnosis rather than to difficulty in operative technique.

Ruptured aneurysms of visceral arteries originally were recognized only as abdominal catastrophes, and survival rates were low. Aneurysms are presented for elective operation infrequently after diagnosis is made fortuitously by angiography. Hepatic artery aneurysms have been resected successfully; methods of preservation of hepatic function must be considered. Splenic artery aneurysms are recognized on angiograms far more often than they are excised. Splenectomy is done, not restoration of continuity. Gastric artery aneurysms have been recognized as causes of intraperitoneal bleeding. Surgical treatment of aneurysms of superior or inferior mesenteric arteries have been reported in small numbers.

RENAL ARTERIES

Reconstruction operations for stenoses of renal arteries in 627 patients caused mortality in 7 percent, and reduced systemic hypertension in 86 percent at one year; 57 percent of patients were normotensive. Smaller series reported from other centers disclosed similar results, 15 to 25 percent of patients not being benefited by operation.

Improved renal function (i.e., glomerular filtration, natriuresis, diuresis, reduced osmolality) follows corrective renal artery surgery. This is vitally important in patients whose ischemic cause of renal failure was life threatening.

ABDOMINAL AORTA

Aneurysms. Of 3,000 patients with abdominal aneurysms, 92 percent survived operation. Only a fraction of this series had been operated upon five and ten years earlier, but survival was 58 percent and 30 percent respectively, at these times. This is a significant improvement over the mortality at five and ten years in 130 patients with abdominal aortic aneurysms observed in the era before incision and graft was possible. Recently Varco and his co-workers[44] questioned the need to excise all aneurysms, citing 16 percent operative mortality versus five year survival rates of 30 percent in patients not subjected to operation. Two other series[43,46] cite far superior results of excision, irrespective of age. Voorhees[47] reported consistently low operative mortality in aneurysmectomy when performed by or under the supervision of experienced surgeons. This was in contrast with a ten-fold increase in morbidity and mortality in a smaller series of aneurysms which had been excised in the same university hospital by competent general surgeons less experienced in vascular surgery.

AORTA-ILIAC OCCLUSIVE DISEASE

Ninety-eight percent of 3,000 patients survived operative correction of stenoses and occlusion of aorta and iliac arteries. Ninety-six percent had immediate restoration of blood flow, which was maintained over the long term in 94 percent. In the young, aged 36 to 45, Najafi[51] reported one-third asymptomatic, one-third symptomatic, and the final third dead at five years following treatment by endarterectomy and reconstruction.

FEMORAL ARTERIES

Aneurysms. The localization of a process in a readily accessible area between large arteries contributed to the acceptably low mortality (3 percent of 440 patients reported by DeBakey[63]) attending excision of femoral artery aneurysms. Postoperative complications within one and two years were bilateral recurrent femoral artery aneurysms which developed between the distal edge of the onlay cloth patch and the presumably incompletely excised aneurysm. Thrombosis developed in one aneurysm, precipitating hospital admission, excision of false aneurysm, thrombectomy proximally and distally, and restoration of luminal continuity with another segment of prosthetic graft.

Occlusive Disease. Seventy-five percent of 2,500 bypass graft operations between femoral and popliteal arteries were patent at one year (DeBakey[72]). Edwards[60] reported progressively improved statistics as experience increased and techniques changed. Long-term patency was achieved in 25 percent with cloth grafts, 65 percent with endarterectomy, and 90 percent with saphenous vein autografts. Connolly and Stemmer[57] reported high patency with in-situ saphenous bypass grafts. Dundas[59] of Oslo reported long-term patency rates, to seven years, at least 10 percent better than femoro-popliteal patency recorded by others. His in-situ technique included excision of valves with resuturing of veins. Blaisdell[56] believed that creation of a temporary arteriovenous shunt improved patency rates in patients with inadequate run-off. Wylie and co-workers[61] and Bernhard, Ellison, and their associates[79] found prognostic significance in blood flow studies performed at operation. Blaisdell[56] reports angiography contributes significantly to higher patency rates early and late.

POPLITEAL ARTERIES

Aneurysms. Wallace and co-workers of the Mayo Clinic reported 31 percent complications in untreated popliteal artery aneurysms.[76] Most surgeons agree now that exclusion and bypass is as useful a procedure as excision, with fewer complications.

ARTERIES DISTAL TO THE KNEE

It is commonplace to terminate reconstruction or bypass procedures distal to the knee with a high degree of early success and long-term patency. Bypass operations to the ankle and beyond have had early operative success around 75 percent, with one-year patency in excess of 50 percent. Obviously, salvage has been a principal indication for these extended risk procedures. Combinations of precise microsurgical techniques, low platelet stickiness, and treatment of synthetic material with wall-bonded heparin, hold promise for high long-term patency rates.

BIBLIOGRAPHY

CAROTID ARTERY

1. CLAUSS, R. H., HASS, W. K., and RANSOHOFF, J. Simplified method of monitoring adequacy of brain oxygenation during carotid artery surgery. *New Eng. J. Med.,* 273:1127, 1966.
2. COTEV, S., LEE, J., and SEVERINGHAUS, J. W. The effects of acetazolamide on cerebral blood flow and cerebral tissue Po_2. *Anesthesiology,* 29:471, 1968.
3. DEBAKEY, M. E., et al. Cerebral arterial insufficiency: One to 11 year results following arterial reconstruction operation. *Ann. Surg.* 161:921, 1965.
4. FRENCH, L. A., and GALICICH, J. H. The use of steroids for control of cerebral edema. W. H. Mosberg, Jr., et al., eds. *In Clinical Neurosurgery, Vol. 10. Proceedings of the Congress of Neurological Surgeons, Houston, Texas, 1962.* Baltimore, The Williams & Wilkins Co., 1964.

5. KETY, S. S., and SCHMIDT, C. F. The effects of altered arterial tensions of carbon dioxide and oxygen on cerebral blood flow and cerebral oxygen consumption of normal young men. *J. Clin. Invest.*, 27:484, 1948.

6. LYONS, C., LELAND, C. C., JR., MacDOWELL, H., and MacARTHUR, K. Cerebral venous oxygen content during carotid thrombintimectomy. *Ann. Surg.*, 89:307, 1964.

7. MOORE, W. S., and HALL, A. D. Importance of emboli from carotid bifurcation in pathogenesis of cerebral ischemic attacks. *Arch. Surg.*, 101:708, 1970.

8. RAINER, W. G., McCRORY, C. B., and FEILER, E. M. Surgery on the carotid artery with cervical block anesthesia. *Amer. J. Surg.*, 112:703, 1966.

9. SIEKERT, R. G., and WHISNANT, J. P., eds. *Cerebral Vascular Diseases: Transactions of the Sixth Conference.* New York, Grune & Stratton, Inc., 1968.

10. VIANCOS, J. G., SECHZER, P. H., KEATS, A. S., and DeBAKEY, M. E. Internal jugular venous oxygen tension as an index of cerebral blood flow during carotid endarterectomy. *Circulation,* 34:875, 1966.

11. VonRUDEN, W. J., BLAISDELL, F. W., HALL, A. D., and THOMAS, A. N. Multiple arterial stenoses: Effect on blood flow. *Arch. Surg.*, 89:307, 1964.

12. WELLS, B. A., KEATS, A. B., and COOLEY, D. A. Increased tolerance to cerebral ischemia produced by general anesthesia during temporary carotid occlusion. *Surgery,* 54:216, 1963.

13. WHITE, C. W., JR., ALLARDE, R. R., and MacDOWELL, H. A. Anesthetic management for carotid artery surgery. *J.A.M.A.*, 202:1023, 1967.

14. YASARGIL, M. G., KRAYENBUHL, H. A., and JACOBSON, J. H. II. Microneurosurgical arterial reconstruction. *Surgery,* 67:221, 1970.

SUBCLAVIAN ARTERY—BRANCHES

15. BAIRD, J. R., and LAJOS, T. Z. Emboli to the arm. *Ann. Surg.*, 160:905, 1964.

16. DALE, W. A., and LEWIS, M. R. Management of ischemia of the hand and fingers. *Surgery,* 67:62, 1970.

17. GONZALEZ, L., WEINTRAUB, R. A., WIOT, J. F., and LEWIS, C. Retrograde vertebral artery blood flow: A normal phenomenon. *Radiology,* 82:211, 1964.

18. MANSFIELD, P. B., GAZZANIGA, A. B., and LITWIN, S. B. Management of arterial injuries related to cardiac catheterization in children and young adults. *Circulation,* 42:501, 1970.

19. RAINER, W. G., QUIANZON, E. P., LIGGETT, M. S., NEWBY, J. P., and BLOOMQUIST, C. D. Surgical considerations in the treatment of vertebrobasilar arterial insufficiency. *Amer. J. Surg.*, 120:594, 1970.

20. SOLTI, F., ISKUM, M., PAPP, S., TURBOK, E., and NAGY, J. The regulation of cerebral blood circulation in subclavian steal syndrome. *Circulation,* 42:1185, 1970.

21. THORENS, S. Arteriosclerotic aneurysms of hand. Excision and restoration of continuity. *Arch. Surg.*, 92:937, 1966.

CORONARY ARTERIES

22. American College of Chest Physicians. *Diseases of the Chest.* Symposium No. 1, August, 1970.

23. BAILEY, C. P., MAY, A., and LEMMON, W. M. Survival after coronary endarterectomy in man. *J.A.M.A.*, 164:641, 1957.

24. EFFLER, D. B., SONES, F. M., FAVALORO, R., and GROVES, L. K. Coronary endarterectomy with patch-graft reconstruction. *Ann. Surg.*, 162:590, 1965.

25. FAVALORO, R. G., EFFLER, D. B., GROVES, L. K., SONES, F. M., JR., and FERGUSSON, D. J. G. Myocardial revascularization by internal mammary artery implant procedures. *J. Thorac. Cardiovasc. Surg.*, 54:359, 1967.

109. Chase, N. E., Hass, W. K., Ransohoff, J. Modified method for percutaneous brachial angiography. *Arch. Neurol.*, 8:632, 1963.

110. Crawford, E. S., DeBakey, M. E., Morris, G. C., Jr., and Howell, J. F. Surgical treatment of occlusion of the innominate common carotid and subclavian arteries: A ten-year experience. *Surgery,* 65:17, 1969.

111. Etheredge, S. N. A simple technic for carotid endarterectomy. *Amer. J. Surg.,* 120:275, 1970.

112. Thompson, J. E., Austin, D. J., and Patman, R. D. Carotid endarterectomy for cerebrovascular insufficiency. *Ann. Surg.,* 172:663, 1970.

113. Yasargil, M. G., Krayenbuhl, H. A., and Jacobson, J. H. II. Microneurosurgical arterial reconstruction. *Surgery,* 67:221, 1970.

CHAPTER 5

OTHER SURGICAL MEASURES

SYMPATHECTOMY
INDIRECT REVASCULARIZATION OF
   MYOCARDIUM
REDUCED WORK OF THE HEART
PARA-ARTERIAL DECOMPRESSION

LOCAL TREATMENT OF NECROSIS

DEBRIDEMENT
INCISION AND DRAINAGE
SKIN GRAFTS
AMPUTATION

PHYSIOLOGIC FITNESS

SYMPATHECTOMY

Sympathectomy (lumbar, dorsal, cervical, splanchnic) is intended to reduce physiologic tonus of arterioles, thereby increasing blood flow regionally. Initially perfusion of blood to the skin is increased, but subsequently this may be negated by sensitivity of vessels to endogenous catecholamines. Perfusion of blood to muscles is not increased; it usually is decreased following sympathectomy.

SELECTION OF PATIENT FOR LUMBAR SYMPATHECTOMY VERSUS RECONSTRUCTION

Marked improvement following endarterectomy, bypass graft, or sympathectomy may be anticipated in patients with abundant large collateral vessels bridging a site of stenosis or occlusion in the superficial femoral artery. Symptoms may be claudication after walking several blocks in the course of normal activities associated with the pursuit of livelihood. The indication for any operation in such a patient is relative, and this is to be understood by the surgeon, internist, patient, and his family. Failure of direct arterial surgery in such ideal circumstances is rare in experienced hands, but it does occur. Lumbar sympathectomy has many proponents here, for a variety of reasons—fear of failure of arterial reconstruction (perhaps undue leaning upon the Hippocratic principle of "first do no harm"), ease and speed of lumbar sympathectomy, and paucity of postoperative care compared to that required after arterial reconstruction. It would appear that only "raw" data of early and late mortality and amputation is of value in the reported clinical follow-up series of patients subjected to sympathectomy. Mortality and amputation rates are said to be low. The quality and duration of relief defies accurate description. Angiographic findings at intervals after all procedures would give a truer picture, but rarely are these findings published. Blood flow studies following sympathectomy cite liabilities of the procedure and contrast unfavorably with flow studies after reconstruction which overwhelmingly support the latter procedure. Many surgeons combine arterial reconstruction with sympathectomy anticipating relief of symptoms of untreated obstructions in distal arteries or increased flow through the corrected segment. This practice too easily dismisses the ill-effects of sympathectomy, and fails to recognize the benefits of reconstruction only.

Stenotic and occlusive lesions demonstrate characteristic patterns angiographically, permitting forecast of end-results of sympathectomy and of direct arterial surgery. This spectrum varies: only gross misfortune should cause failure in ideal cases, where lesions are segmental and usually confined to the superficial femoral artery. In contrast, a near-miracle would be required to relieve claudication with sympathectomy or to maintain patency in some arteries with high-grade stenoses distributed diffusely in the popliteal-tibial system. Operation in the favorable category may be advised as a luxury to free patients of discomfort, permitting greater latitude in work or recreation. Operative repair of vessels with diffuse and extensive occlusions is reserved as an alternative to major amputation (e.g., ischemic lesions of threatened or actual gangrene, infection difficult to control, intolerable rest pain). The record of sympathectomy in providing symptomatic improvement or limb salvage in these instances not only is not impressive, but sympathectomy may be contraindicated here.

Extensive thrombosis or arterioarterial emboli rarely are spontaneous complications of high-grade stenoses of superficial femoral arteries, but they may be avoidable by reconstructive operation prior to complication. Every experienced surgeon at times has found occluded vessels which appeared patent on angiograms a few days earlier. Progression of symptoms during hospitalization and despite anticoagulation therapy has been observed. Doubtless, similar thrombotic episodes may explain reported instances of rapid progression of symptoms or gangrene following sympathectomy.

Sympathectomy may seem to have a place in improving circulation to the skin in patients with threatened necrosis, especially after failure of direct arterial reconstruction. Alternative nonsurgical measures (dibenzyline, heparin) may be equally effective initially and afford more long-term benefit. Angiographic studies of limbs unsuited for reconstruction and amputated after failure of treatment with phenoxybenzamine and reflex vasodilation by heat uniformly disclose recent occlusions not apparent on earlier angiograms.

No relief may be anticipated following sympathectomy in microvascular diseases, where there is markedly abnormal morphology and flow through small vessels 7 to 30 µ in diameter, and undue sympathetic tonus is not the problem. Clinical diagnosis may be suspected by history and findings (Chapter 3). Capillary microscopy is important to establish the diagnosis and to quantify the extent of abnormality.

Wesolowski[11] presented a plea for sympathectomy in the treatment of frostbite, but without classification of capillaroscopic findings.

CERVICAL SYMPATHECTOMY

Upper extremity.   The rarity of atherosclerotic occlusion of arteries of the upper extremity limits the need to choose between nonsurgical measures, sympathectomy, and arterial reconstruction. Thus, ischemic findings in upper extremities obligates consideration of microvessel diseases as causes of symptoms in hands and arms. Capillaroscopy is a passive diagnostic test for the patient and *can* be diagnostic. Angiography can delineate local atherosclerotic processes amenable to reconstruction or disclose typical tapering patterns of microangiitis requiring treatment of the basic disease. Antiadrenergic drugs may effect considerable measures of relief to vasospastic conditions, and sympathectomy is rarely required.

Carotid-vertebral arteries.   Chemical or surgical ablation of the cervical sympathetic ganglia or of the chemoreceptor bodies of the carotid bifurcation do not increase blood flow to the brain directly. Prevention of hypersensitive reflex phenomena which cause bradycardia and hypotension may be effected by adventitial stripping of the carotid sinus.

Coronary arteries.   Interruption of pain pathways is possible by infiltration of the cervical plexus and the first and second thoracic sympathetic ganglia with local anesthesia. Neurectomy, once a popular procedure, is no longer performed.

Celiac mesenteric or renal arteries.   Denervation of these arteries is not performed to relieve ischemic symptoms of viscera.

LOCAL DENERVATION

Denervation of major blood vessels by stripping adventitia from them appears unreasonable in this decade of angiography and vascular reconstruction. Physiologic understanding of the role and limitations of effects of nerves upon circulation and knowledge of increasingly precise sites of actions of drugs make denervation an unnecessary procedure.

Neurotomy had transient and limited popularity. Its current appeal despite rare practice is that sensory denervation relieves pain; regional sympathectomy is effected, and skin circulation may be improved. It bears repeating that angiography can disclose the limitations of local blood supply and thus the impracticality of the procedure (neurotomy) in most instances.

Local infiltration of focal areas of pain (and presumed ischemia) in calf muscle sites is advocated by some surgeons.

INDIRECT REVASCULARIZATION OF MYOCARDIUM

Arterial implant into myocardium has achieved respectable status in selected instances, when demonstrated stenoses greater than 90 percent have been followed by angiographic evidence of patency of implant and communications between implant and intrinsic coronary vasculature in 80 percent of patients.

Deepicardialization with phenol or mechanical techniques has relieved pain and has led to increased myocardial collateral circulation.

Coronary venous obstruction increased collateral circulation in experimental animals. Clinical use of this has been abandoned.

Counterpulsation is a technique whereby extracorporeal apparatus increases diastolic pressure and flow to coronary arteries.

Reduced Work of the Heart

Reduced cardiac contractility secondary to decreased metabolic rate reduces oxygen requirement.

β-adrenergic blockade (propranolol) decreases ventricular contractile force, rate, and abnormal rhythms.

Results of all indirect techniques are not dramatic, except where sensory nerves are ablated, and are less than satisfactory when basic arterial disease is too advanced to permit appreciable increase in flow in response to the procedure employed.

Para-Arterial Decompression

Exhaustive treatises exist regarding symptoms, signs, diagnostic maneuvers, and management of subclavian artery compression by scalenus anticus muscle hypertrophy, cervical rib, or clavicle. External compression of celiac axis by crus of diaphragm and narrowing of femoral artery by adductor tendon have been reported relieved by operation. The hazards of encasement of cloth grafts in scar tissue are believed to be fixation leading to kinking during flexion. The authors have observed external compression of vein grafts within weeks of reconstructive operations. Diminished pulse and defect on angiogram have precipitated exploratory and corrective operations. Careful operative hemostasis and purposeful drainage of wounds appear necessary to minimize hazards of scarring.

TREATMENT OF NECROSIS AND INFECTION SECONDARY TO ISCHEMIA AND/OR DIABETES MELLITUS

Debridement

CONTRAINDICATIONS—"FIRST DO NO HARM"

Dry gangrene describes ischemic necrosis without apparent infection. The involved skin or part is discolored, usually blue-black, and painless. Distal phalanx or entire toes may be involved. The process frequently seems spontaneous, yet pressure of shoes or bedclothes may have been sufficiently compressive to exclude circulation to involved areas long enough to cause death of tissue. Necrosis of the skin of the heel or over the bony prominence of the metatarsal or malleolus commonly is ascribed to pressure. Tissue death probably involves skin first, then deeper layers. Local operation is to be avoided unless testing (v.i.) indicates regional circulation is adequate for healing. Successful revascularization of major arterial pathways may need to be accomplished before local healing is assured.

Autoamputation of digits can occur. Spontaneous healing of necroses over heel, malleolus, and metatarsal head is not common, for at these sites autoamputation cannot occur.

Local operation is never to be done as a trial of adequacy of circulation, or with unsubstantiated hope of healing after limited, unwarranted excision, when blatant contraindications to operation exist. These are pain at rest, inflammation and/or edema across the intended line of transection, or venous filling time greater than 20 seconds.

INDICATIONS

Wet gangrene implies infection. Stages of wet gangrene are edema, serous transudate becoming purulent exudate, and gradations of extent, depth, and virulence of infection and its necrotic consequences. A bulla may become contaminated, then infected. A fissure may excite an exudate separating layers of skin. Deep fissures admit contamination to subcutaneous tissue; spread may proceed into and along tendon sheaths or joint capsules and joints. Cartilage and bone may become involved, the former dying, the latter capable of periosteal reaction defensively.

Treatment should look immediately to the procedure that will result in healing, namely surgical excision of the infected joint and bones. Patients generally are not markedly febrile and there is not lymphangitis. Initial therapy for 24 to 48 hours consists of systemic antibiotics, bed rest, slight elevation of the part, painless excision of the scar and superficial necrotic tissue to assure unroofing of the wound, and instructions for the patient to lie in a lateral or prone position if necessary to promote drainage. Smear and culture of exudate is obtained before instituting gram-positive and gram-negative coverage with antibiotics. Ampicillin, 500 mg three times a day before meals and a fourth time before bedtime, generally is ample initial antibiotic therapy. Rigorous attention is given to control of diabetes mellitus. Angiography may be performed the day after admission, for there generally is not lymphangitis, and if there is, the catheter may be introduced into the arterial system from the opposite side. If one elects to perform a local femoral artery injection, this is permissible, and no instances of suppuration of inguinal nodes or disruption of the femoral artery have occurred following femoral puncture on the side affected with lymphangitis. By the second day in the hospital, diabetes is generally controlled well enough to anticipate operation. Both arterial reconstruction and distal local excision of infected parts may be performed at the same operation.

Undrained infection may progress. Thrombosis in small vessels may be induced by bacterial infection. Metabolic demand of infectious processes may divert blood flow from nearby parts; edema may separate capillaries from nutrient-dependent tissues. Nonetheless, in addition to systemic administration of antibiotics, local infected processes require removal of *all* dead tissue. The novice learns the rule of the seasoned practitioner: *remove no living tissue*; bleeding or pain indicate that excision has transgressed the bounds of necrosis. Incision or manipulation which crosses local tissue barriers incites further inflammatory reaction, commonly extending necrosis. At times, ill-effects associated with debridement may be inevitable due to the process and merely coincidental with timing of a procedure. For example, unroofing an infected bulla frequently is followed rapidly by full-thickness necrosis.

Enzyme debridement might be ideal if its application were controlled. As used, it rarely is confined to necrotic sites, and it appears to macerate non-necrotic tissues. Applied to tissues with dry gangrene, barriers to entrance of infection appear disrupted resulting in wet gangrene. Enzyme debridement should not be used in lieu of indicated mechanical removal of tissue, for the latter can be prompt and near total, effecting needed drainage at once.

INCISION AND DRAINAGE

The purpose of incision into loculated purulent tissue is to initiate drainage; the latter must continue until healing occurs or definitive measures are taken. The process of drainage is aided by mechanical separation of parts by cloth, rubber, or plastic materials. Gauze introduced into wounds has specific purposes: compression (hemostasis), absorption, and gross removal of debris. "Packing" is a misnomer which perpetuates bad habits; the term is inconsistent with good concepts.

Excision of both viable and nonviable tissue (radical debridement, amputation) is acceptable only when local circulation is adequate for primary or secondary healing. There are instances when such open amputations must be done immediately, to remove the source of continuous emission of toxic products into the body. Primary closure is contraindicated in the presence of gross contamination. Major bleeding points are controlled with minimal amounts of fine

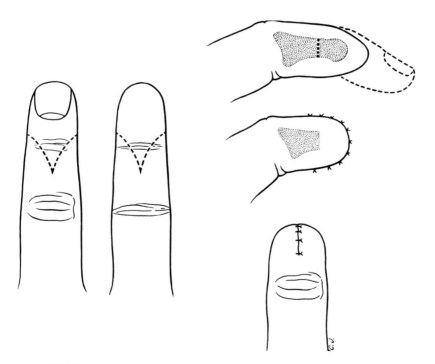

Figure 5-1. BIVALVE SKIN FLAPS, with bases formed laterally on neurovascular pedicles heal so well there is no discomfort from the supple, hairline scar.

absorbable or monofilament nonabsorbable ligature, and the wound surface is covered with telfa, against which sufficient gauze is placed to provide pressure to stop bleeding and bulk to absorb drainage.

Racquet incision has been conventional and has the apparent merit of dependent drainage. In truth, needed drainage is achieved by periodic assumption of a prone position by the patients. Excision of toes through phalanges may be performed satisfactorily with flaps of equal size based laterally (Fig. 5-1). Digital arteries nourish these flaps well.

Tendons and tendon sheaths are cleanly incised at the proximal limits of the amputation site. No attempt is made to draw the tendon into the wound for excision and retraction. This is likely to leave dead space for accumulation of contaminated debris.

When hemostasis is effected by adequate or excessive pressure, it follows that some packing must be removed soon, to preclude necrosis from inadequate circulation. Incorrectly, a wound commonly is stuffed to its capacity. Excess packing is withdrawn without removing material in direct contact with tissue. Subsequently, dressings must serve as drains, not stoppers. Absorptive characteristics of cloth drains remove exudate, the pablum for bacteria. Wet packing is ineffective for absorption. Thus, moisture determines the frequency of changing dressings; once a day may not be often enough. The base of a wound should cease to appear purulent within 12 to 48 hours if debridement was adequate, if systemic antibiotic therapy is effective, and if further circulatory failure has not occurred. Diminished size (capacity) of a wound is expected as granulation tissue grows, and edema subsides. Among the most common ill-effects of excess packing is the prevention of contraction, cicatrization, and granulation.

Irrigation, soaking, dependent drainage, or mechanical cleansing eliminate the need for drains or packs in wounds in which the skin edges do not coapt spontaneously before the base closes by contraction and tissue growth. Continuous soaking is contraindicated for it macerates intact skin, making it vulnerable to infection. Rarely should wound care be made the province of nurses. Attentive physicians can act upon observations that individual (not routine) care encourages. The need to alter technique, antibiotics, or operation is likely to be detected and acted upon sooner. Judgment becomes mature; interest and innovation yield better care, quicker healing, or earlier decision regarding definitive treatment.

Excision of a metatarsal-phalangeal joint is readily accomplished with epidural, spinal, or general anesthesia. It is important to excise infected bone and all cartilage of the joint (Fig. 5-2). It is equally important to avoid entering the contiguous joint, which is easy when excising the fifth metatarsal-phalangeal joint, as it is well proximal to the fourth joint, or the first, separated sufficiently from the second. However, the fourth, third, and second metatarsal-phalangeal joints are virtually side-by-side, and if excision of these joints is done, it is imperative to examine the x-ray to have a clear idea of the contiguity of the joints, so that an adjacent joint space is not entered. The first and fifth metatarsal-phalangeal joints may be excised, leaving the toes in continuity with the foot. However, when two or more contiguous joints are removed, blood supply to the outermost toe is jeopardized, and it is probably wise to excise toes to prevent secondary necrosis. The amount of skin that is removed from plantar and dorsal aspects when joint

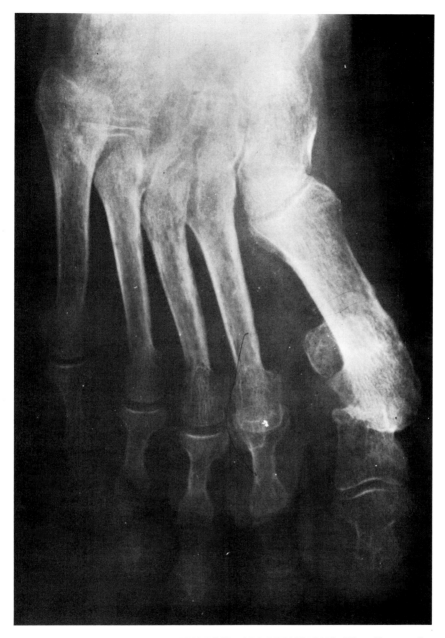

Figure 5-2. ANATOMY OF METATARSAL AMPUTATIONS. The distance between first and second metatarsal heads allows amputation free of danger of inadvertent entry into joint space of second metatarsal-phalangeal joint. (Infection destroyed first m-p joint in this photograph.) Lateral separation and proximal location of fifth m-p joint facilitates amputation of fifth metatarsal. Clustering of heads of second, third, and fourth metatarsals enhances danger of unintentional operative injury or entry into adjacent joint space during amputation. Such injury is avoided by deliberate incision into mid-point of m-p joint of digit being excised, leaving intact the lateral aspects of this joint capsule.

and toes are excised is an amount that permits the flaps to fall together to close the wound while avoiding redundancy. Excess distal tissue can perform no useful function.

AVOIDABLE ERRORS OF LOCAL CARE OF ISCHEMIC EXTREMITIES

It is important not to miss the diagnosis, when a patient presents himself early, before x-ray evidence of destruction of the joint is apparent, but when gentle probing will disclose infection into the joint. Excision at this time removes the lateral portion of the capsule and all the cartilage. Little bone need be removed. It is important to realize that long-term antibiotic treatment is unlikely to effect sterilization of the joint and cartilage and healing of the wound. Whether the osteochondritis and osteomyelitis are recognized or not, it is important not to be exhaustive in antimicrobial laboratory workup and didactic approach. An experienced surgeon will not whittle away pieces of a patient prior to major amputation. Experienced physicians will not inflict morbidity by vain attempts to achieve, with a long period of medical therapy, what is unlikely to be attained, and what can and should be accomplished quickly with a localized surgical operation.

The usual criteria for assessing likelihood of healing of distal incisions are applicable. If inflammation is contiguous with the wound (and does not cross the site of intended incision) and venous filling time is less than 20 seconds, almost certainly the wound will heal properly.

Care following local excision of infected tissues involves drainage for the first few days, followed specifically by removal of packing to permit the skin edges to fall together and the wound to contract and heal. This process is rapid between the third and sixth days, and it is important to avoid mechanical separation of wound parts at this time.

Skin Grafts

Split-thickness skin grafts may be applied immediately after excision of the necrotic base of an ulcer of the heel, malleolus, or metatarso-phalangeal joint. These grafts should be sutured to the wound edges. There is virtue in a dressing designed to absorb transudate. It may be preferable to protect but not cover skin grafts.

Pinch grafts are disadvantageous because of greater thickness and subtotal covering of wound.

Healing ("take") of skin grafts may be affected by the amount of fibrosis in the base of wounds. Fibrosis tends to increase with duration of existence of the ulcer. Longstanding lesions may require excision of their base to remove the fibrous barrier to circulation.

Amputations

It is an accepted principle that angiograms must precede amputations, minor or major. Clinical guidelines of the level of amputation are specific. High morbidity and mortality of amputations continue unchanged, due to serious disease in aged patients, failure to heed the lessons of the past in selection and infection. Failure of primary healing occurs in 25 to 40 percent of below-knee amputations, 10 percent of above-knee amputations. Mortality is 10 percent for below-knee amputations, 25 to 40 for those above the knee. A corollary of these warnings of sequelae of amputation is that advanced age and serious co-existing diseases are not absolute contraindications for arterial reconstruction. Soft-tissue operations elicit far less systemic stress response than amputations.

AMPUTATION, IMMEDIATE FITTING, AND EARLY AMBULATION

The psychologic trauma of major amputation may be lessened by immediate fitting of a prosthesis. Physical debility may be minimized by early ambulation.

Patients frequently are bedridden for weeks in attempts to salvage extremities. Then, with psyche, physical strength, and financial resources at low ebb, amputation is a major imposition. However, the seemingly unbearable prospects of disability can be made acceptable to patients and their families. A patient may be told about immediate fitting of a prosthesis shortly before amputation and wake from anesthesia to find that a painful, life-threatening disability has been exchanged for a prosthetic limb. This he can see is a new source of hope. Patients stand the day after amputation. Walking, supporting weight, use of parallel bars, and touching the prosthesis to the ground, follow within a week. Crutch walking begins by the tenth day. Weight-bearing proceeds by the end of the second week. The gait becomes normal by the end of the third week, and patients may leave the hospital at this time. Young, vigorous patients whose limbs have been amputated for trauma or tumor frequently walk unassisted by the end of the third week. The aging patient with amputation for ischemic atherosclerosis and/or diabetes generally is self-supporting on a prosthesis without crutches in six to eight weeks.

A review of the routine course of patients with major amputations at Bellevue Hospital disclosed that seven months elapsed before amputees were self-sufficient on prostheses.[7] A review of the literature in a selected series of below-knee amputations, in which early ambulation was the goal, disclosed that walking could be effected in eight weeks.[6]

The concept of early fitting and ambulation has employed certain technical features which have improved the quality of amputations. Weiss[10] of Poland believes that proprioception is retained when fascia of amputated muscles is attached to periosteum of bone. Essential afferent and efferent stimuli are transmitted and appropriate motion of the extremity is effected because muscles are shortened (lengths commensurate with level of bone) and secured to bone. Varieties of major modifications of surgical techniques employ the basic idea of fixation of fascia. In above-knee amputations, anchoring fascia of anterior and posterior, and lateral and medial musculofascial groups to bone, covered by medial fixation of fascia lata, creates a stump of ideal size and optimal function. Below-knee amputations employ the gastrocnemius muscle and its tendon, suturing the latter to the fascia of the anterior aspect of the tibia, creating a weight-bearing muscle pad over the ends of both bones. The soleus usually is excised, and the fibula is amputated 1.5 inches shorter than the tibia. Skin flaps are made with a longer posterior flap.

Drainage is not employed. Collodion or telfa and one gauze dressing are applied to the closed wound, followed by one sterile stockinette, and one stump sock pulled over the amputation wound and onto the proximal thigh. Padding is placed to protect the tibial tubercle, head of fibula, and patella in below-knee amputations. No padding is needed in above-knee amputations. Elastic plaster of paris dressing is rolled virtually skin tight. When the knee is flexed ten degrees, the below-knee cast is self-retaining. Straps incorporated into the cast of above-knee amputation stumps retain the cast by a belt or over-the-shoulder suspension arrangement.

Weiss[10] has reported the use of continuous drainage for 48 hours, followed by partial opening of cast and removal of drain. We have not used drainage, and stumps have healed well. Necrosis has not been observed when casts were removed after three weeks. Casts dislodged or removed within two weeks of amputation at times disclose 15 to 30 cc of serous material beneath skin flaps which can be removed by aspiration. In some instances of removal of casts two weeks after amputation, necrosis up to several centimeters in diameter has occurred, generally along the anterior flap. The prosthesis may be reapplied and ambulation continued. Dressings are changed as needed, and the necrotic area sloughs, granulates, cicatrizes, and heals. Despite failure of primary healing, with its infection, drainage, and closure by secondary intention, more people leave the hospital earlier walking on a prosthesis than was observed when regimens did not include early ambulation.

PHYSIOLOGIC FITNESS

Assessment of cardiac response to activity is equally applicable to amputees, athletes, and astronauts. Much that was learned from extensive careful observation of the latter applies to the ill, inactive, or aged patient. Undue increase in heart rate in response to increments in activity is to be interpreted as a warning of unsuitability for that level of activity.

Deconditioning is a term applied to the "softness" incurred by inactivity. Reconditioning commonly requires twice the period of time of inactivity. If a healthy youth at bed rest for three weeks manifests tachycardia after resumption of "normal activity," it is expected that the aged subject has far less reserve. When bedridden patients are made to sit, stand, or walk, heart rates over 100, or rises of 20 above resting rate, are likely to occur and commonly are associated with giddiness and/or hypotension. Activity is discontinued at once, and graded exercises in prone or recumbent positions are instituted to recondition patients to prepare them to stand and to walk.

Observations of cardiac output and oxygen cost of routine activities show surprising multiples of resting levels in response to standing and walking. How much greater, then, is the burden of an untrained septuagenarian-turned-athlete as he struggles with balance and bars, pain and prosthesis!

The common practice of placing at bed rest a patient with ischemic complications of an extremity must be accompanied with conditioning exercises. The old practice of Buerger's exercises (see Chap. 6, p. 181) may have had general systemic conditioning as its principal virtue. Reflex activity of nerves of the venous system occur with lowering an extremity. Arbitrary resumption of the excessive activity of early ambulation must be tempered with awareness of the importance of preventive observations to preclude myocardial damage. Tachycardia may be secondary to hypovolemia, maldistribution of body fluids, or inadequate myocardial capacity. Most patients respond quickly to retraining. The physician and therapist must monitor heart rate as one of the best guides to patients' capacities for work.

BIBLIOGRAPHY

1. Boyd, A. M. The role of sympathectomy in the management of intermittent claudication. *Vasc. Dis.*, 3:137, 1968

2. Eastcott, H. H. G. *Arterial Surgery*. Philadelphia, J. B. Lippincott Co., 1969.

3. Haimovici, H., Hoffert, P. W., Zinicola, N., and Steinman, C. An experimental and clinical evaluation of grafts in the venous system. *Surg. Gynec. Obstet.*, 131:1173, 1970.

4. Hawthorne, H. R., ed.: *Vascular Surgery*. Springfield, Ill., Charles C Thomas, Publisher, 1965.

5. Harrison, C. E., Jr., Spittell, J. A., Jr., and Mankin, H. R. Sudden arterial occlusion: A clue of silent myocardial infarction. *Mayo Clin. Proc.*, 37:293, 1962.

6. Hoar, C. S., Jr., and Torres, J. Evaluation of below-knee amputation in treatment of diabetic gangrene. *New Eng. J. Med.*, 266:440, 1962.

7. Russek, A. Personal communication.

8. Sako, Y., and Varco, R. L. Arteriovenous fistula: Results of management. *Surgery*, 67:40, 1970.

9. Vaughan, B. F., Slavotinek, A. H., and Jepson, R. P. Edema of the lower limb after vascular operations. *Surg. Gynec. Obstet.*, 131:282, 1970.

10. Weiss, A., Gidinski, A., and Wirski, J. Myoplasty—immediate fitting and ambulation. Reprint of Paper presented at World Commission on Research and Rehabilitation. Wiesbaden, Germany, 1966.

11. Wesolowski, S. A., et al. The role of sympathectomy in frostbite with a review of 68 cases. *Surgery*, 57:774, 1965.

12. Wheelock, F. C., Jr. Transmetatarsal amputations and arterial surgery in diabetic patients. *New Eng. J. Med.*, 264:316, 1961.

CHAPTER 6

MEDICAL MANAGEMENT

ARTERIAL SYSTEM

PHYSIOLOGIC MEASURES
PHARMACOLOGIC MEASURES
  Antilipid Drugs
  Vasoactive Drugs
  Anticoagulant Drugs

Fibrinolytic Agents
Dextran

MANAGEMENT OF UNDERLYING AND
  ASSOCIATED CONDITIONS

MICROCHANNELS

ARTERIAL SYSTEM

PHYSIOLOGIC MEASURES

Medical management of patients after operative restoration of primary arterial channels is directed toward general preventive and supportive measures. Dietary advice, regulation of habits (including occupational adjustments when necessary), and treatment and management of underlying or associated conditions are intended to improve the length and quality of survival.

It is widely accepted that obese people have a higher incidence of mortality from cardiovascular disease than nonobese persons. It appears mandatory to maintain patients' weights 10 percent below "normal" standards of insurance companies by regulating carbohydrate intake. Diets low in saturated fat are prescribed for patients with occlusive arterial disease due to atherosclerosis.

Smoking is not a desirable habit for patients with arterial disease, as it affects blood flow and arterial wall lesions. Nicotine increases the amount of circulating catecholamines, and in those who are sensitive to it nicotine causes diminution of blood flow to skin. Nicotine has been shown to increase lipemia; thus, the possibility of enhancement of atheromatous disease by smoking is evident. The higher incidence of coronary atherosclerosis in smokers is well documented.

Medical treatment to enhance collateral circulation is directed not only to lessening vasomotor tone but also to preventing further vasoconstrictor impulses to the area. The basic principles of a peripheral vascular routine have been generally accepted, and the following measures may be recommended:

Keep extremities dry and warm (avoid cold).

Avoid injuries.

Encourage vasodilation with heat (reflex, not local), exercise, and alcohol ingestion.

An important point in such daily measures is to shield carefully the afflicted part against injury of any kind. Wide, firm shoes which accommodate as many pairs of woolen socks as necessary are advisable. The patient and a member of the family are to examine toes and feet daily for fissures and discoloration and to report them immediately to the doctor. All directly applied physiotherapeutic procedures (e.g., local heat, contrast temperature baths) must be avoided.

Applying heating pads to flanks for one hour twice a day, and remaining warm and in bed a second hour, induces release of tonus in vessels. Carefully graded exercise under supervision is done according to a flexible plan; quantitation of daily increments is based on repeated clinical evaluation. Reflex heat and graded exercises independently act to increase blood supply to the extremity and to improve the vasomotor responses in the limb. One ounce of Scotch, bourbon, or brandy three times a day has a salutary anticonstrictor effect. Much has been written about correlations between smoking and coronary artery disease, elevation of catecholamine concentrations and of lipid levels in blood. In thromboangiitis obliterans and other types of angiitis possibly due to tobacco sensitivity there is an indisputable direct correlation between smoking and progression of the disease; these patients have to give up tobacco unconditionally to keep their limbs.

Patients confined to bed may conveniently take graded exercises in the form of the well-known Buerger's exercises, performed several times daily for half an hour each time. The following sequence is recommended: The patient, lying on his back, first places his feet on a support that provides an elevation of about 25 cm (10 inches) for one minute and flexes his toes and feet rhythmically; following that, he sits up at the edge of the bed and dangles his feet for one minute. One minute of rest in the horizontal position completes the cycle. This should be repeated ten times, according to the patient's general status. It is advisable to permit these patients dependency of the affected limbs to about 5 to 10 cm below the horizontal for at least a few hours each day, unless edema formation prohibits this. For patients whose general status (chronic congestive heart failure, severe chronic pulmonary failure, extensive ulcerations, debilitations, etc.) excludes even the use of Buerger's exercises, the Saunders oscillating bed may be used to induce rhythmic changes of blood volume and hydrostatic pressure in the extremities and centrally. Heart failure is associated with peripheral vasoconstriction. Postural decompression of central circulation simultaneously supplies a greater hydrostatic pressure gradient to peripheral arteries.

PHARMACOLOGIC MEASURES

ANTILIPID THERAPY

The use of some well-tolerated thyroid preparation may be a desirable adjunct for patients with documented hypercholesterolemia. In some types of hyperlipemia, especially those connected with mild hypothyroidism in the elderly, Choloxin in doses of 4 to 8 mg daily has proved effective. The effects upon vascular disease of long-term use of the new cholesterol-depressant medication remains to be determined. In carbohydrate-induced hyperlipemia, notably that connected with diabetes mellitus, Atromid-S (clofibrate) in doses of 1000 to 3000 mg daily considerably lowers the lipid concentration in the blood. Braunwald, et al.[17] have found that reactive hyperemic responses in the lower limbs of man are improved by the administration of Atromid-S.

There has been an increasing tendency to try to increase collateral arterial blood supply by using drugs, usually designated as vasodilators. In recent years, many drugs capable of inducing vasodilation in various vascular beds have been developed. The reports on their pharmacologic qualities have stimulated renewed interest in the possibilities of medicinal treatment of hypertensive disease as well as of periphral vascular disase. When a new drug is being evaluated, patients are likely to benefit psychologically from the increased attention they receive. Without objective measurements, it is difficult to be certain that the new agent under study truly is effective, or whether patients' stimulated attentiveness to cleanliness, careful dressing of ulcers, and physical methods (reflex dilation and graded exercise) have contributed to clinical improvement.

It appears convenient to classify drugs that affect extremity blood flow according to their measurable physiologic sites, modes, degrees, and limitations of actions in man and according to pharmacologic chemistry. An important and voluminous literature is accumulating correlating these mechanisms of action.

ADRENERGIC STIMULATION. Epinephrine markedly increases blood flow to the skeletal muscles, while decreasing blood flow to the skin. Several epinephrine-related compounds have a marked vasodilator effect on resting muscle, and even more so on working skeletal muscle, while the constrictor effect on skin vasculature seems to be minimized. The clinical results in the treatment of intermittent claudication are not as impressive as the experimental results seem to suggest. However, in the absence of major trophic changes in the skin, these drugs appear to be indicated in treatment of intermittent claudication not correctable by vascular reconstruction. Arlidin (nylidrin HCl) and Vasodilan (isoxuprine HCl) are the most widely used. Their side-effects are increased myocardial irritability, as expressed in the appearance or aggravation of extrasystolic arrhythmias and (rarely) aggravation of preexisting anginal syndrome. Recently an experimental drug, bamethan sulfate, has been developed, which seems to excite fewer cardiac side-effects

ADRENERGIC BLOCKADE. The predominant action of Dibenzyline (phenoxybenzamine), a close relative of Dibenamine, is on the vessels of the skin. In addition to its antiadrenergic action, there is some evidence that the drug may also have a direct action on vascular musculature. Dibenzyline given orally over long periods of time increases blood flow to the extremities in normal individuals as well as in patients with marked arteriosclerosis obliterans and Buerger's disease. Dibenzyline has a wide range of effective dosage and tolerance. Vasodilatation of vessels of the extremities can usually be obtained without causing disabling hypotension. It has seemed to us at times that the more extensive the organic vascular disease, the higher the tolerated dose. For example, a patient with far-advanced obliterative endoarteritis tolerated and required 400 mg daily to secure vasodilation. Ilidar (azapetine phosphate) can also be used over long periods of time and may be given orally. Increased blood flow to the lower extremities has been documented plethysmographically and by surface temperature recordings.

The side-effects of adrenergic blocking—stuffiness of nose and throat and fixation of pupil—are usually present to a mild degree but, although unpleasant, are not serious side-effects. It must be noted that this drug is contraindicated in asthmatic patients because of the congestion of the upper respiratory passages which accompanies its use. Giddiness and listlessness induced by hypotension or tachycardia have been bothersome in some cases. Tachycardia is a frequent and serious side-effect which sometimes may be avoided by simultaneous administration of reserpine. Hypotension is to be avoided for the possibility of its dreaded effects. Another side-effect of Dibenzyline may be failure of ejaculation during sexual intercourse. This is in contrast to the impotence which develops in patients being treated with ganglionic blocking agents. All these so-called complications are actually direct sequelae of complete adrenergic blockade. Agents whose action is on the ganglia have not been practical in the treatment of peripheral vascular disease because hypotension almost invariably develops.

Considerable success has been achieved with Dibenzyline in the treatment of gangrenous ulcers which were progressing at such a rate that amputation was being considered. Often relief of pain was dramatic and prompt; of greater importance, these gangrenous ulcers began to heal slowly. First, demarcation of the border of gangrene became clear, and then healing began. The degree of relief of intermittent claudication was less impressive and very slow.

A combination of Dibenzyline orally and use of enzymes (Varidase) locally for digestion of necrotic material has been used. The maximal effect of Dibenzyline alone on the rate of healing of ulcers may be increased by the use of Varidase; similarly, the maximal rate of healing in response to use of the enzymes can be increased by administration of Dibenzyline. When Dibenzyline and Varidase have been used simultaneously, healing of gangrenous ulcers has seemed to take place more rapidly. More important than the speed of healing, however, is that healing has been completed by the combined use of these two agents when neither agent alone seemed effective.

ANTICOAGULANT DRUGS

Anticoagulants can effectively decrease the danger of embolization from peripheral venous thrombosis as well as from intracardiac thrombi. Their long-term use in chronic rheumatic heart disease, especially before and after cardiac surgery, seems well justified. Stasis and thrombogenic surfaces virtually demand induced alterations in coagulability to obviate thrombus formation.

Various interpretations have been accorded the published data of large series of patients with myocardial infarction treated with long-term anticoagulation therapy. In some cases, namely those liable to develop intracardiac or venous thrombi (e.g., failure, cardiac dilatation, arrhythmias, peripheral circulatory disturbances), the use of anticoagulants for one or two years seems justified, based on the same rationale. Comparable data may never be possible, since angiographic survey, assessment of platelet stickiness, and hematologic and lipid profiles appear to be required for true comparability.

There is no evidence to suggest that anticoagulants are of any value in occlusive arterial disease. In cerebral as well as in peripheral manifestations of occlusive atherosclerosis, their uselessness is well established. We have had occasion to document the development of occlusive atherosclerosis in a large number of patients with atherosclerotic heart disease who have been kept on a long-term anticoagulation program following myocardial infarctions.

FIBRINOLYTIC AGENTS

Fibrinolysis as a therapeutic measure in recently established vascular thrombosis is theoretically attractive. Streptokinase is widely used in Europe, and urokinase is undergoing extensive clinical trial in this country. However, none of the clinical studies reported is sufficiently well controlled to warrant convincing conclusions. The supply of urokinase is limited and available only to a few investigators.

DEXTRAN

Concepts and facts of electric charge upon vessel walls and platelets have encouraged therapy which may alter surface charges and clotting propensities. Low molecular weight dextran has been employed with favorable consequences in experimental preparations conducive to arterial thrombogenesis. Clinical application of Macrodex 70 (high molecular weight dextran, not dextran 40) in preventing venous thrombosis compels attention; statistically significant prevention of thrombophlebitis in patients with fractured hip treated by nailing was obtained by Nilsson and co-workers,[2] infusing 500 ml of Macrodex 70 daily for three days, and every third day thereafter. All patients were subjected to phlebography. The incidence of phlebitis was reduced from 50 percent in untreated patients to 4 percent. No bleeding complications occurred.

The relation between degrees of platelet adhesiveness, thrombus formation, and thromboembolic disease appears to become more firmly established as ease, standardization, and reliability of techniques have encouraged wider investigation. The high correlation between increased platelet adhesiveness and early thrombosis of arterial reconstructions contrasts with prolonged high patency rates in patients with normal or subnormal platelet adherence to test surfaces. Aspirin, Persantine (dipyridamole), Robitussin (sulfinpyrazone), pyridinolcarbamate, and altered plasma protein (e.g., by dextran) appear to exert favorable antiadherence effects by decreasing the numbers of young platelets or, in the instance of dextran, by altering the interaction between platelets and collagen of surfaces of vascular wall or grafts.

MANAGEMENT OF UNDERLYING AND ASSOCIATED CONDITIONS

Atherosclerotic heart disease is present in almost all patients with occlusive atherosclerotic disease of the extremities. These patients must be carefully observed and treated for their cardiac needs. The strain of pain, secondary infection, and progressive gangrene in extremities often have deleterious effects on the cardiac status. The manifestations of ischemic heart disease, including old myocardial infarction, are by no means contraindications to vascular surgery.

Diabetes mellitus may adversely influence the course of vascular disease in two ways. Microvessel disease emerges as a contributing factor of the diabetic disease syndrome. This small vessel disease seems to affect small arteries, such as the digital arteries, much more frequently in diabetics, and it is not uncommon to find gangrene of one or several toes in the presence of perfectly perfused dorsalis pedis and posterior tibial vessels. Secondary infection is more difficult to control than in the nondiabetic patient. These ill effects of diabetes mellitus are ameliorated in well-controlled diabetic carbohydrate metabolism. Whenever dietetic measures do not suffice, insulin is preferred to the oral hypoglycemic agents. It has not been proved conclusively that the islands of Langerhans contribute to the mechanism of action of oral hypoglycemic agents, whereas the majority of diabetics do have hypoinsulinism. It is recognized that hypoproduction of insulin is not the only cause of the diabetic disturbance, but it certainly is one of its major aspects, and insulin is the specific physiologic replacement therapy.

In long-term illness, oral administration of a drug is of first importance because other modes of administration tend to disrupt the individual's way of life. Intramuscular administration is next in preference because the patient can be taught to use this method at home. Intravenous and intra-arterial injections are inconvenient, as they require the patient's attendance at a clinic or office or require medical personnel to visit the patient's home. Long duration of action of drugs is highly desirable. Unpleasant or dangerous side actions must be avoided.

MICROCHANNELS

Remission or effects of treatment of basic disease processes simultaneously improves microangiitis. Stated another way, therapeutic measures for recognized diseases of minute vessels are identical with those effective in the management of the basic disease entities (e.g., connective tissue diseases, hematologic disorders, immunologic disorders, diabetes mellitus). Ulcerations due to minute vessel diseases (microthrombi?) usually heal with remission of the basic disease or in response to treatment with corticosteroids and/or infusion of low molecular weight (40,000) dextran.

The therapeutic approach to pathologic changes in minute vessels and to disturbances in blood flow through these channels is being explored by several groups of workers. Treatment aligns along three pathways: corticosteroids, alpha-lytic drugs, and low molecular weight dextran.

CORTICOSTEROIDS

In connective tissue disease, the responses of the microvessels to corticosteroids are dose-dependent. There is an individual optimum dosage level *at* which microangiitic manifestations are minimized (ulcers heal, livedo reticularis diminishes) but *below* or *above* which these manifestations are exaggerated. Discontinuing treatment may preciptate ulceration and gangrene.

ALPHA-LYTIC DRUGS

An abnormal sensitivity to catecholamines may be the basis of some form of microangiitis. For example, capillaroscopy discloses marked narrowing of the afferent limb associated with enormous widening of the efferent limb in progressive systemic sclerosis, in various grades of scleroderma. This has led to the trial use of alpha-lytic drugs, such as guanethidine and phenoxybenzamine. Given in small doses, their effects (e.g., on Raynaud's phenomenon) sometimes are striking. The side-effects (e.g., lowering of systemic arterial pressure, tachycardia, provocation of anginal syndrome) call for extreme caution.

LOW MOLECULAR WEIGHT DEXTRAN

It is possible to combat the most striking rheologic sign of microangiitis (increased intraluminal aggregates) by changing the molecular milieu of the blood. Low weight molecular dextran (Swedish rheomacrodex, molecular weight 40,000) has been used to treat progressive systemic sclerosis and to enhance healing of microangiitic ulcerations.

Further development of therapy for microangiitis is dependent upon recognition and definition of basic pathologic microcirculatory patterns and their gradual integration with known circulatory, metabolic, and hematologic disease entities.

To date, there is no agent capable of demonstrably repairing damage to the capillary wall or predictably influencing capillary permeability.

Symptoms arising from regulatory disturbances in the minute circulation may be relieved considerably with the use of pharmacologic agents of the nicotinic acid group. Thus, physiotherapeutic measures, especially contrast baths (alternate immersion of the extremity in warm water for two minutes and cold water for one minute), may be helpful. In chronic trenchfoot, microvessel tone has been lost and clumps of cells impede circulation. Dilatation with drugs or warmth allows movement and dissipation of these aggregates; transiently induced constriction may propel the circulation.

BIBLIOGRAPHY

1. ABBOUD, F. M., et al.: Preliminary observations on the use of intra-arterial reserpine in Raynaud's phenomenon. *Circulation,* 36 (Suppl. 2):49, 1967.
2. AHLBERG, A., NYLANDER, G., ROBERTSON, B., CRONBERG, S. and NILSSON, I. M. Dextran in prophylaxis of thrombosis in fractures of the hip. *Acta Chir. Scand., Suppl.* 387:83, 1967.
3. BAUER, J. *Differential Diagnosis of Internal Diseases.* New York, Grune & Stratton, Inc., 1967.

4. BRADSHAW, P., and CASEY, E. Outcome of medically treated stroke associated with stenosis or occlusion of the internal carotid artery. *Brit. Med. J.*, 1:201, 1967.

5. BUCHWALD, H., MOORE, R. B., FRANTZ, I. D., JR., and VARCO, R. L. Cholesterol reduction by partial ileal bypass in a pediatric population. *Surgery*, 68:1101, 1970.

6. DEPALMA, R. G., HUBAY, C. A., INSULL, W., JR., ROBINSON, A. V., and HARTMAN, P. H. Progression and regression of experimental atherosclerosis. *Surg. Gynec. Obstet.*, 131:633, 1970.

7. FOLEY, W. T. Treatment of gangrene of the feet and legs by walking. *Circulation*, 15:689, 1957.

8. GOODMAN, L. S., and GILMAN, A. *The Pharmacologic Basis of Therapeutics.* New York, The Macmillan Company, 1970.

9. LEHR, D. Tissue electrolyte alteration in disseminated myocardial necrosis. *Ann. N. Y. Acad. Sci.*, 156:344, 1969.

10. RAAB, W. *Preventive Myocardiology.* Springfield, Ill., Charles C Thomas, Publisher, 1970.

11. REDISCH, W. Tobacco allergy and vascular responses. *In* James and Rosenthal, et al., eds. *Tobacco and Health.* Springfield, Ill., Charles C Thomas, Publisher, 1962, pp. 352*ff.*

12. ——— The relationship between diabetes and obliterative arteriosclerosis. Selected papers from symposia and training conferences on diabetes mellitus. N. J. State Dept. of Health, Div. Chronic Illness Control, Diabetes Control Program, Diab. DI, pp. 16*ff*, July, 1961.

13. ——— Peripheral vascular disease. *In* Covalt, D. A., ed. *Rehabilitation in Industry.* New York, Grune & Stratton, Inc., 1958.

14. ROMEO, S. G., WHALEN, R. E., and TENDALL, J. P. Intraarterial administration of reserpine. *Arch. Intern. Med.*, 125:825, 1970.

15. WELCH, C. C., et al. Cinecoronary arteriography in young men. *Circulation*, 42:647, 1970.

16. WRIGHT, I. S. Recent developments in antithrombotic therapy. *Ann. Intern. Med.*, 71:823, 1969.

17. ZELIS, R., MASON, D. T., BRAUNWALD, E., and LEVY, R. I. Effects of hyperlipoproteinemias and their treatment on the peripheral circulation. *J. Clin. Invest.*, 49:1007, 1970.

EPILOGUE

The scientific knowledge and technical advances of our time, admirable as they are, can best fulfill their purposes of easing the burdens of human existence when directed by mature humanistic spirit and wisdom. The great humanists were universally educated and oriented. The solution to arterial disease must be preventive through more complete understanding. Considering atherosclerosis and coronary heart disease, dare one predict that fuller comprehension may permit unrestricted enjoyment of diet, activity, and environment without ill-effect? Today's vast and ever-increasing accumulation of information precludes universality of knowledge in individuals, but teamwork and interdisciplinary integration can herald the revival of universality. Currently, while those with symptomatic atherosclerosis must be considered highly susceptible, are they perhaps fortunate to be identified "at risk" of further consequences? The calculated use of the best of knowledge, applied with a perspective of (not *by*) one physician to solve the unique problems of single patients, may fulfill the "new look" in universal humanism.

INDEX